COMMUNITY HEALTH AND WELLNESS NEEDS ASSESSMENT
A Step-by-Step Guide

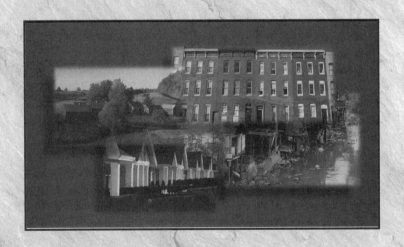

COMMUNITY HEALTH AND WELLNESS NEEDS ASSESSMENT
A *Step-by-Step Guide*

Editors

Deena A. Nardi, PhD, APRN, BC, FAAN
College of Nursing and Health Professions
Lewis University, Romeoville, Illinois

Josy M. Petr, MS, RN
Indiana University School of Nursing
Indiana University Northwest

THOMSON
™
DELMAR LEARNING

Australia · Canada · Mexico · Singapore · Spain · United Kingdom · United States

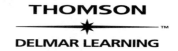

THOMSON

DELMAR LEARNING

Community Health and Wellness Needs Assessment: A Step-by-Step Guide
Edited by Deena A. Nardi, PhD, APRN, BC, FAAN and Josy M. Petr, MS, RN

**Executive Director,
Health Care Business Unit:**
William Brottmiller

Executive Editor:
Cathy L. Esperti

Acquisitions Editor:
Matthew Filimonor

Senior Developmental Editor:
Marah Bellegarde

Editorial Assistant:
Patricia Osborn

Executive Marketing Manager:
Dawn F. Gerrain

Channel Manager:
Jennifer McAvey

Project Editor:
Mary Ellen Cox

Production Coordinator:
Anne Sherman

Art/Design Coordinator:
Robert Plante

Library of Congress
Cataloging-in-Publication Data
Community health and wellness needs assessment: a step-by-step guide / [edited] by Deena Alleria Nardi, Josy Petr; contributing authors, Charlene Gyurko . . . [et al.].
    p. ; cm.
    Includes bibliographical references and index.
    ISBN 0-7668-3498-0 (alk. paper)
    1. Community health services.
    2. Needs assessment. I. Nardi, Deena Alleria. II. Petr, Josy.
    III. Gyurko, Charlene.
    [DNLM: 1. Community Health Services. 2. Health Promotion.
    3. Needs Assessment.
    WA 546.1 C73355 2003]
    RA427 .C616 2003
    362.12—dc21   2002025602

NOTICE TO THE READER

CONTENTS IN BRIEF

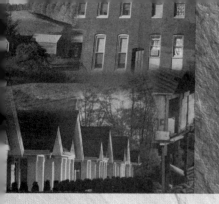

CONTENTS

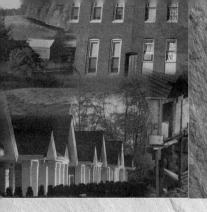

PREFACE
Josy M. Petr

This guide is designed for individuals and groups involved in comunity health promotion activities such as grant proposal writing, project development, program funding, and policy promotion. It is also designed as a supplemental book to be used by students of various disciplines in courses where they will learn the essential concepts of conducting a community health and wellness needs assessment. Students can also use it as a resource following their graduation and transition into practice.

Any individual or group can design, develop, and implement a health and wellness needs assessment for any population, in a short period of time, regardless of funding available to them, if the participants:

- have the motivation to do the work
- are invested in the work
- and have a plan that includes strategies for obtaining and evaluating results

This book is a step-by-step guide to doing the work of conducting a health and wellness needs assessment of any population, including minorities, homeless, underserved, uninsured, aging, and rural. It can be used as a tool, providing a plan that can be clearly articulated and easily understood by all who would like to be able to first assess health and wellness needs before planning interventions to promote health.

WHY WE WROTE THIS BOOK

The authors were part of a group at a Midwest university who collaborated with members of their community to conduct an assessment of the health and wellness needs of three local counties as a first step in the development of service and research proposals. They were surprised to discover that many health care and human services providers were unaware of existing data that could be accessed quickly, easily, and inexpensively. Also, they were convinced that students, health care providers, practitioners, community leaders, and other professionals would benefit from an easy-to-use, step-by-step guide to conducting a comprehensive health and wellness needs assessment. The authors' purpose is to share their tool. The intent is not to present a comprehensive guide for the uses of various models. Instead, the authors intend to describe, in detail, the model they developed, how they used it, and how it might be easily used by others.

CONCEPTUAL APPROACH

This unique book presents a step-by-step guide to a process model for conducting a health and wellness needs assessment that is based on the Ontario Needs Impact Based Model, the World Health Organization definition of health, *Healthy People 2010* goals, and secondary analysis of existing data. In each chapter, examples of uses of this model are provided that will assist others in learning the application of this process so that they can conduct their own community health and wellness needs assessment. The assessment is tied to *Healthy People 2010* goals, which in turn become the benchmarks for health and wellness needs identification and program achievements.

Four elements contribute to the process model and the usability of this book. These include Ontario Needs Impact Based Model, WHO Definition of Health, *Healthy People 2010,* and secondary analysis of existing data.

Ontario Needs Impact Based Model

The framework presented in this guide is based upon the Ontario Needs Impact Based Model. It is transtheoretical, not dependent on one particular community health theory, and can be used as a framework by any health and human services discipline in any community or situation. This model integrates needs assessment, prioritization, program planning, and evaluation and conducts needs assessment in four steps:

1. Definition and description of the needs assessment problem
2. Determining what information is required
3. Information gathering
4. Analysis of the information

Throughout the process, a broad definition of health and wellness is used not only to emphasize social factors in the overall determination of the health of the community and its individuals, but also to indicate need.

World Health Organization Definition of Health

In this book, wellness refers to a general satisfaction in all areas of an individual's life, including aesthetic, cultural, educational, emotional, environmental, mental, relational, and spiritual. Health is defined as "a state of complete physical, mental and social wellness and not merely the absence of disease or infirmity" (WHO, 2001, p. 1). The World Health Organization's classic definition of health was chosen for use with the Ontario Needs Impact Based Model because it is holistic, used globally, and broad enough to include social factors such as socioeconomic status, education, safety, and the environment in the overall determination of the health of communities and individuals.

A community assessment project is most often conducted by diverse groups or teams and is guided by a blend of two or more perspectives to meet the objectives of the assessment. The transtheorectical Ontario Needs Impact Based Model, when combined with the World Health Organization definition of health, can be used alone or integrated with other frameworks/models whose goals are to arrive at a holistic view of the community.

Healthy People 2010 Goals as Benchmarks

The *Healthy People 2010* draft document points out that "*Healthy People 2010* is the United States' contribution to the World Health Organization's 'Health for All' strategy" (U.S. Department of Health and Human Services, 1998, Introduction 2). It goes on to describe efforts by the United States as being characterized by the work of collaborative groups with community participation. By using national objectives, the United States provides a model for world policy and strategies for improved population health.

Secondary Analysis of Existing Data

Secondary analysis is used in this book as one method for identifying, gathering, grouping, and analyzing existing data from valid sources. It is most useful when time and financial resources are limited, and is especially helpful for comparing sample characteristics to benchmarks. Methods of inquiry such as focus groups, key informant interviews, and traditional surveys are also described. These qualitative methods can be used with secondary analysis of existing data to illustrate, validate, and enrich data gathered from existing sources.

ORGANIZATION

Chapter 1

The first "how to" chapter introduces health and wellness assessment as a holistic process that encompasses physical, psychological, social, environmental, and economic aspects of life in the United States. The World Health Organization definition of health and *Healthy People 2010* goals and benchmarks for improving heath and wellness are used to define and identify selected areas of health and wellness. This process recognizes needs assessment as the critical first step in health planning. A number of health assessment models that can serve as conceptual frameworks for conducting a health needs assessment are compared to the Ontario Needs Impact Based Model. Secondary analysis of existing data methodology is introduced as the method of choice for conducting relevant and cost-effective community health and wellness needs assessments.

Chapter 2

In the second "how to" chapter, steps of the needs assessment process are described further, beginning with the need to address confidentiality of data and issues of informed consent. Application of the steps is demonstrated using an example of a health assessment question arising from the observations of a single practitioner. This chapter also illustrates the process, application and credibility of secondary analysis of existing documents as a method of needs assessment that is rigorous, cost-effective, and useful in action research studies throughout the nation.

Chapters 3, 4, and 5

The next three chapters focus on examples of applying the steps of the community health and wellness assessment process to three areas of concern:

- ◆ Physical health and wellness
- ◆ Mental health and wellness
- ◆ Maternal, child, and family health and wellness

Each of these chapters introduces factors that are specific to the assessment of these particular domains of heath and wellness. For instance, Chapter 3 uses the OPT model, or outcome-present state-test model of clinical reasoning, to guide assessment of physical health and wellness needs in the community. Chapter 4 examines the legislative and economic variables that have influenced how community mental health support services are organized, funded, and used. Chapter 5 explains the social, physical, and environmental factors that impact the health and degree of wellness of the childbearing family.

At the end of each chapter, a needs assessment tool demonstrates how identified data can be compared with benchmarks to determine the current health and wellness status and current health systems operations of a selected community by using actual data gathered from a tricounty area as a representational sampling. These practice models provide tools for use by nurse educators, the academic community, and public health and service operations to assist in addressing regional health and wellness outcomes.

Although we have standardized presentation of the chapters, we must note that the data and goals presented in Chapters 3, 4, and 5 are very different. We purposely presented each chapter differently to address the issues and problems related to each domain (for instance, for Chapter 3, the interrelationship of diabetes and heart disease can be directly demonstrated, but the interrelationship between addiction and child abuse is more contextual and cannot be directly attributed in Chapter 4).

Chapter 6

Chapter 6 introduces the community-based indicators movement and the capacity of the health care system to provide quality health care to diverse populations in the community.

Chapter 7

Chapter 7 describes the completion of the steps by demonstrating how results can identify the particular health and wellness needs of the community. Findings can be examined for themes or underlying connecting attributes, grouped accordingly, and compared to *Health People 2010* benchmarks to identify health and wellness needs and plan interventions. The results of this analysis can be used to sharpen the focus and increase the usefulness of primary health care programs and institutions.

Chapter 8

Resources presented in this chapter can be used as key indicators, benchmarks, and selected data to assist in developing and conducting a health and wellness needs assessment. Resources here include official state and national documents and web-based materials, as well as studies on key indicators and other health and wellness needs assessment studies.

FEATURES

- Learning objectives help focus reader's attention on pertinent content.

- Key terms are bolded and defined within chapters.

- Many examples to assist others in conducting their own community needs assessment are provided.

- Examples of assessment and analysis of specific data addressing *Healthy People 2010* goals are presented in table form with an explanation of the processes used to solve the assessment problem.

- Resources that include official state and national documents, and web-based materials, as well as studies on key indicators and other health and wellness needs assessment studies, are provided at the conclusion of this text.

- Twenty-eight additional assessment tool tables, one for each *Healthy People 2010* goal, can be downloaded from the Delmar online resources web site @ hitchcock.delmarnursing.com. The 28 tables provide a tool template that all health care providers can use to gather their own data.

OTHER DELMAR LEARNING PRODUCTS

Community Health Nursing: Caring in Action, 2e
Janice Hitchcock, Phyllis Schubert, Sue Thomas
Order # 0-7668-3497-2
A concise, innovative community health nursing textbook, *Community Health Nursing: Caring in Action, 2E* presents all major community and public health topics. This revised edition emphasizes the roles and responsibilities of the community and public health nurse, with special emphasis on international, multicultural, poverty, alternative healing modalities, and other emerging themes. A new full-color design and many photographs and illustrations further help bring this edition to life.

Community Health Nursing Case Study CD-Rom
Janice Hitchcock, Phyllis Schubert, Sue Thomas
Order # 0-7668-3499-9
This CD-Rom presents 20 critical thinking case studies involving community health scenarios. The learner is presented with a scenario and is prompted to answer questions.

Handbook of Community Health Nursing: Tools and Resources
Janice Hitchcock, Phyllis Schubert, Sue Thomas
Order # 1-4018-1273-2
The perfect nurse companion! This handbook presents tools and forms commonly used by community health nurses in an easily portable size.

ABOUT THE AUTHORS

The authors are health and human services educators who teach in the fields of nursing, business, social policy, and child development. They share the belief that health care providers, educators, community leaders, and policy makers must assess a community's health and wellness needs in order to better understand them and their implications for primary health care and human services program development.

 ## REFERENCE

World Health Organization (2001). Definition of health. *About WHO* [on-line]. Available: www.who.int/aboutwho/en/definition.html.

ACKNOWLEDGMENTS

This book would not have been written without the groundwork laid years before by Doris R. Blaney, EdD, RN, FAAN, dean emerita and professor emerita, Indiana University School of Nursing Northwest Campus. Her association with community groups and work with health care professional organizations in Northwest Indiana provided the framework that made possible the regional health and wellness assessment that our group participated in. We are also grateful to the U.S. Department of Health and Human Services for its permission to integrate its *Healthy People 2010* national initiative throughout our step-by-step process.

The authors would like to thank the reviewers of the book for their constructive feedback:

Rebekah Damazo, PHN, PNP, MSN
School of Nursing
California State University
Chico, CA

Linda Hulton, RN, PhD
Assistant Professor of Nursing
James Madison University
Harrisonburg, VA

Virginia Nehring, PhD, RN
Associate Professor, College of
Nursing and Health
Wright State University
Dayton, OH

Rebecca Robinson, PhD, RN
Associate Professor
West Texas A & M University
Canyon, TX

Rachel Spector, PhD, RN
Department of Nursing
Boston College
Boston, MA

INTRODUCTION TO HEALTH AND WELLNESS NEEDS ASSESSMENT

Deena A. Nardi

 LEARNING OBJECTIVES

At the conclusion of this chapter, the reader will be able to:

- ◆ Explain the purpose of a health and wellness needs assessment.
- ◆ Define health and wellness.
- ◆ Explain health assessment models that serve as a conceptual framework for conducting a needs assessment.
- ◆ Describe the steps of conducting a health and wellness needs assessment.
- ◆ Apply secondary analysis of existing data methodology to data identification, gathering, and analysis.
- ◆ Use *Healthy People 2010* determinants of health as focus areas for beginning examination of a community's health and wellness.

▨ KEY TERMS

Action research	Health
Benchmarks	Leading health indicators
Culture	Objectives
Community	Ontario Needs Impact Based Model
Conceptual framework	Secondary analysis of existing data
Determinants of health	Target population
Goals	Wellness

This chapter introduces health and wellness needs assessment as a holistic process that encompasses physical, psychological, social, spiritual, environmental, and economic aspects of life in the United States. The World Health Organization (WHO) definition of health and *Healthy People 2010* goals and benchmarks for improving health and wellness are used to define and identify selected areas of health and wellness. **Goals** are broadly worded focus areas that provide direction for action and guide an assessment. *Healthy People*'s 28 goals, or focus areas, were derived from its two overarching goals (to improve quality and length of life and to eliminate health disparities). This process recognizes needs assessment as the critical first step in health planning. Secondary analysis of existing data is introduced as one method of choice for conducting relevant and cost-effective community health and wellness needs assessments. **Community** refers to groups composed of individuals, families, organizations, or businesses that share a common language, common values, a common history, or a common purpose.

PURPOSE OF A HEALTH AND WELLNESS NEEDS ASSESSMENT

Health is defined using the WHO definition that describes it as a "state of complete physical, mental and social wellness and not merely the absence of disease or infirmity" (WHO, 2001, p. 1). See Box 1-1. This broad definition of health emphasizes the importance of social factors such as socioeconomic status, education, safety, and the environment in the overall determination of the health of the community and the individual. **Wellness** refers to quality of life, a general satisfaction in all of the areas of an individual's life, including aesthetic, cultural, educational, economic, emotional, environmental, mental, physical, relational, and spiritual.

A health and wellness needs assessment can serve as a foundation for improved communication and cooperation within a community or target population in identification of health and wellness service and evaluation needs. A **target population** is a group within a community, or a group within several communities, which shares a given concern or attribute. A needs assessment can also stimulate a greater collaboration between community health care providers and populations within the community, and educational and research institutions and organizations. Identified needs can also serve to provide direction to county Education and Health Departments as they prioritize and deploy their resources. Health and wellness assessments are used to set goals, locate and distribute health and human services resources, set policy, and communicate needs to target populations within the community. Recommendations derived from these assessments provide the framework for working with the community to establish measurable health and wellness goals for its target populations, including the underserved rural, minority, homeless, and low-income pregnant and parenting populations.

A health and wellness needs assessment report about a community or a target population within a community marks the end of the first phase of a project, and the beginning of the next and final phase—the development of research and service-based proposals and projects, and the securing of external funding for both. The end result of these proposals and projects should demonstrate a more concerted effort to address identified health and wellness needs, for target populations and communities, and can contribute to the health and wellness of the community.

> **Box 1-1 ■ World Health Organization Definition of Health**
>
> *"Health is a state of complete physical, mental and social well-being and not merely the absence of disease and infirmity."*
> —*World Health Organization, 2000, p. 1*

HEALTH AND WELLNESS DEFINED

Since 1946, when the newly formed WHO published its classic definition of health in its first Constitution, the nations of the world have steadily adapted that holistic definition for their own use in identifying and addressing their health and wellness needs. The United States has lagged behind other nations in universally adapting the WHO definition (Huq, 1999), partially because its 50 state Departments of Health are semiautonomous, sometimes insular, and not centrally organized. The WHO definition of health is a holistic concept that is a resource for living, and incorporates aesthetic, behavioral, cognitive, economic, educational, environmental, political, psychological, and social factors (World Health Organization, 1986). It is used in this book, however, because it is universally accepted and serves as a global measure of wellness that ties in well with the general goals of *Healthy People 2010*.

The U.S. Department of Health and Human Services (DHHS) has adopted a similar definition of health as inextricably linked to the health and wellness of the community, as well as influencing the overall health of the entire nation. This world view of health and wellness is reflected in its vision statement, "Healthy People in Healthy Communities" (U.S. Department of Health, 2000, p. 1). See Box 1-2.

> **Box 1-2 ▪ Healthy People's Vision of Health**
>
> *"A healthy community is one that embraces the belief that health is more than merely an absence of disease; a healthy community includes those elements that enable people to maintain a high quality of life and productivity"*
>
> — *U.S. Department of Health, 2000, p. 1*

CONCEPTUAL BASIS FOR CONDUCTING A COMMUNITY HEALTH AND WELLNESS NEEDS ASSESSMENT

There are a number of health needs assessment models that serve as **conceptual frameworks** for conducting a health needs assessment. Conceptual frameworks are developed to explain the relationships between concepts and between concepts and a phenomenon to be studied. They provide guidelines for understanding what is known about the phenomenon and what needs to be known about it (Nieswiadomy, 2002). The health needs assessment models presented here hold in common the tenet that health care and health seeking behaviors are influenced by multiple factors. These assessment models provide a point of view from which to prioritize and direct an assessment, identify pertinent issues, and determine which data sources to use. A selection of the most common categories of theoretical models is presented here and summarized in Table 1-1.

TABLE 1-1 Common Categories of Theoretical Models

MODEL	DESCRIPTION	USE IN NEEDS ASSESSMENT
Community-as-Partner	Community is target of and partner in assessment. Community consists of a core of people and eight subsystems.	Includes assessment of core and all eight subsystems.
Ecological	Health and wellness are affected by multiple levels of environmental influences that occur at individual, interpersonal, organizational, community, and public policy levels.	Determines the influence of environment on health and wellness behaviors, as well as the influence of these behaviors on the environment.
Health Behavior	Consumers' uses of health services is determined by their perceptions of threats to health and benefit of using services, plus triggers that cause them to seek services.	Helpful in predicting use of existing health services. Examines health knowledge, psychomotor capacities, and self-management skills.
Health Belief	Focus is consumers' beliefs about the efficacy of health behaviors and practices, and their relationship to the consumers' use of health services.	Often used to explain and predict primary health behaviors for the prevention of illness, disease, and other health conditions. Useful in guiding development programs that provide incentives for consumers to use services, and act on their own behalf.

The Community-as-Partner Model

The community-as-partner model was first termed the "community-as-client model" as an illustration of the key public health role of nursing (Anderson & McFarlane, 2000). This model focuses on the community as the target of and the partner in health needs assessment. The community is considered the expert in determining its needs. Health care providers form collaborative partnerships to empower communities to identify their own health issues and develop their strategies. This model presents the community as consisting first of a core of people who create the community, and focuses on their values, beliefs, history, and pertinent demographics. Eight subsystems—the physical environment, community safety, transportation, health and human services, economics, education, politics and government, and recreation—interact with the core in a transactional relationship that affects both the core and these subsystems. Assessment of the community's health and wellness needs must include an assessment of this core and all eight subsystems as well. Establishing a partnership between health and wellness service providers and the community core is key to accurate assessment, planning, implementation, and evaluation of any health services (Shellman, 2000).

Ecological Models of Health Behavior and Health Promotion

Ecological models of health behavior and health promotion have been used since the nineteenth century in the United States to study the public's health. Their basic principle is that health and wellness are multifaceted, and are affected by multiple levels of environmental influences that range from the natural environmental domain (i.e., the location, weather, and pollution) to the constructed environmental domain, such as home, work, school, social, and recreational environments (Stokols, 1992). These environmental influences occur at the individual, interpersonal, organizational, community, and public policy levels (Perry, Williams, Mortenson, Toomey, Komro, Anstine, McGovern, Finnegan, Forster, Wagenaar, & Wolfson, 1996). Individuals actively shape their health and wellness through an ongoing process of micro- and macro-regulations (Bronfenbrenner, 1979; Garbarino, 1990). If applied to health and wellness behaviors, assessments are directed at determining the influence of the environment on behaviors, as well as the reciprocal influence of these behaviors on the surrounding environment. This model is used to assess health and wellness needs at multiple levels, in order to determine the various levels of influence from environmental factors on discrete health and wellness outcomes, such as those described in *Healthy People 2010* (U.S. Department of Health and Human Services, 2000).

Health Behavior Models

Health behavior models view health services as dependent on several factors that can be grouped into three domains:

1. The consumer's preference for and inclination to use health services.
2. The consumer's need for such health services.
3. The presence of enabling factors that facilitate the consumer's access to and use of such health services. Enabling factors can include such variables as age, gender roles and expectations, culture, race, ethnic group, socioeconomic status, educational level, employment status, and motivation. **Culture** refers to a pattern of values, beliefs, and behaviors that a population or group demonstrates. This cultural pattern will influence how a target population views and values health and wellness, and how it accesses and uses health and wellness services. These enabling factors will also interact with the three components of health behavior models.

Components of health behavior models are health knowledge, psychomotor capacities, and self-management skills (Anderson & Newman, 1973; Aday & Anderson, 1974). In other words, consumers' use of health services is determined by their perception of the threat to their health, their perception of the benefit of these services, and triggers that cue them to seek services. There are several types of health behavior models, used generally to guide studies of health behavior change. These models can be clustered into models of individual, interpersonal, group, and community change, and are useful in predicting use of existing health services.

Health Belief Models

The term "health belief model" is sometimes used interchangeably with "health behavior model." These models are often used to explain and predict primary health behaviors for the prevention of illness, disease, and other health conditions (Jane & Becker, 1984). Their focus is on consumers' beliefs about the efficacy of their health behaviors and health practices, and their relationship to the consumers' use of health services. Health belief models are influenced by the social psychology theory of Kurt Lewin (Hothersall, 1995). They propose that consumers assess their susceptibility to a disease or health condition and the risks involved, and weigh the costs and benefits involved in seeking preventive health services. Triggering factors that influence consumers' health seeking behaviors include access to health services, the consumers' and their significant others' perceptions of the problem, and the effectiveness of their usual home care remedies (Rosenstock, 1990). These models are useful in guiding the development of health education programs that will provide incentives for consumer use of services, and that seek to empower consumers to take action competently on their own behalf.

Ontario Needs Impact Based Model

The Ontario Needs Impact Based Model is a process model that provides a conceptual framework for planning a needs assessment. It is a transtheoretical model that was designed to be used by a multidisciplinary group for assessing diverse target populations. It provides a conceptual framework that integrates needs assessment, prioritization, program planning, and evaluation. It was initially developed by the Ontario Ministry of Health using the framework created by the Canadian Institute for Health Information (Heale, Webster, & Abernathy, 1996). This model conducts needs assessment in four steps: (1) definition and description of the needs assessment problem; (2) determining what information is required; (3) information gathering; and (4) analysis of the information (Heale & Abernathy, 2000). A definition of health and wellness is used throughout the process to indicate need. This definition is broad enough to emphasize the importance of social factors such as socioeconomic status, education, safety, and the environment in the overall determination of the health of the community and the individual. The Ontario model was chosen as the vehicle for demonstrating the process of health and wellness needs assessment in this book, because it is not dependent upon one particular community health theory, but allows for integration of various theories for purposes of needs assessment planning. It can thus be used as a framework for conducting assessments in any health and human services discipline and in diverse communities or situations.

Recommendations for research/evaluation also use the definition of **action research**, or participatory research incorporating community service. This is appropriate to the missions of most health care educational institutions, which prepare their graduates to address real problems in the real-world situations of their communities. O'Brien (1998) defines action research as that which "aims to contribute both to the practical concerns of people in an immediate problematic situation and to further the goals of social science simultaneously. Thus, there is a dual commitment in action research to study a system and concurrently to collaborate with members of the system in changing it in what is together regarded as a desirable direction. Accomplishing this twin goal requires the active collaboration of researcher and client, and thus it stresses the importance of co-learning as a primary aspect of the research process" (p. 2). Simply put, researchers are involved in addressing community problems as they contribute to the well-being of the community they are studying.

HEALTH NEEDS ASSESSMENT PROCESS METHODS

Health needs assessment requires the use of an organized procedure to identify, gather, examine, and analyze the data of interest to the group. The following five methods are the most common for conducting a needs assessment:

1. Focus groups
2. Interviews with key informants
3. Traditional survey methodology
4. Secondary analysis of existing data
5. Geographic information systems

Focus Groups

Focus groups are often used to assess the health and wellness needs of specific constituencies, such as senior citizens in a community or members of a certain faith-based organization. A focus group involves an interview with a small, homogeneous group of individuals, usually community members, using open-ended questions. Open-ended questions are questions that cannot be answered by one- or two-word statements, but require personal reflection, consideration, and a verbal response reflecting the individuals' beliefs, feelings, or thoughts about the subject in question. Focus groups are used to provide qualitative insights into topics that cannot be derived from most written questionnaires (Patton, 1990). Focus groups usually consist of six to nine individuals, and last from one to two hours. They are not discussion groups; the interviewer asks a series of questions in order to gain an understanding or focus political action. Focus groups can be held at any time during the needs assessment process. The traditional focus group consists of a small group of users who discuss issues and concerns, guided by a moderator. The discussion is recorded, sometimes on videotape, and is then analyzed. In health needs assessment, the best use of a focus group is to determine the expressed and felt needs and wants of members of a specific community.

Interviews with Key Informants

Interviews with key informants, who are recognized as having experience or expertise with a specific issue, can provide valuable information and insights into the needs of a community or a specific group within the community (Polit & Hungler, 1997). A key informant is a community

leader with a religious, academic, criminal justice, education, health, or political background, who meets the criteria for inclusion in the assessment.
A semistructured interview questionnaire, or an interview guided by an
outline (Wilson, 1993), is commonly used to guide questions and encourage key informants to share personal perspectives and experiences.
After the interview, the key informant is asked to recommend anyone that
the interviewer should talk to, who meets the criteria for inclusion in the
assessment. This step is part of a "snowball" sampling technique (Trachim,
2000), which allows the interviewer to maximize the number of information-rich key informants over a short period of time. The snowball of key
informants becomes exponentially bigger as the interviewees name other
key informants. Eventually, the same informants will be named by several
sources, which indicates that the interviewer has reached data redundancy
and it is time to conclude this method of data gathering (Patton, 1990).

Traditional Survey Methodology

Traditional survey methodology can be used to study any population,
large or small. Surveys use data gathered from a small sample, which represents the larger population that is to be studied (Wilson, 1993). To be
credible, however, the sampling technique must be rigorous, and must follow procedures determined and understood beforehand by everyone involved in the study. This procedure begins with identifying the research
problem, defining terms, and outlining and maintaining the gathering,
analysis, and interpretation of the data (Kerlinger & Lee, 2000). Data gathering is usually done through the use of an interview schedule, or an outline of questions to be asked by the interviewer. Surveys can be done by
phone, Internet, mail, or personal interview. They are commonly used in
social sciences and in health care to determine the expressed, normative,
felt, and comparative needs of specific population groups (Schutt, 2001).

Secondary Analysis of Existing Data

Secondary analysis of existing data and analysis of public records are
methods of identifying, gathering, grouping, and analyzing existing data
from valid sources such as the U.S. Census Bureau and the U.S. Department of Health and Human Services. Secondary analysis of existing data
is a commonly used method of inquiry in the social sciences (Graves,
1998). Other sources used to analyze existing data are population statistics,
morbidity and mortality statistics, other health surveys and major data
sources, and reports of health risk behaviors in a region, a state, or nation-

ally. Focus groups and individual interviews with selected key members of health advocacy and health provider groups can be used to describe, illustrate, validate, and enrich the data gathered from these sources. Secondary data analysis is especially useful for comparing sample characteristics, for operating under a reduced lead time, and for conducting assessments under financial constraints, since it is a relatively inexpensive application of health informatics.

All research methodology has its limitations, and secondary analysis is no exception. The researcher must be aware of the limitations and take steps to identify, address, and compensate for them. In this case, secondary analysis of existing data uses data that is archived or referred to in some secondary fashion, and is a commonly accepted form of inquiry. However, as with all modes of inquiry, it comes with its own set of limitations and caveats. Every study is conducted with a specific purpose in mind and a set of circumstances at hand, which can influence data gathering and analysis, interpretation, and application of the results. Therefore, secondary analysis must be conducted carefully, always considering the possible biases and differences that can render comparison, or extrapolation to a larger data set, meaningless. To avoid this occurrence, all data should be extracted from valid sources, such as the Department of Health and Human Services, and be closely evaluated. To facilitate application of the data presented, complete references should be used, which enables the reader to access the following information for each item of discrete data: study source, purpose, setting, research design and method, sampling criteria, operational definitions, known biases, and limitations of the primary study data.

Members of the assessment team must not have been on any of the primary research teams to avoid influencing the interpretation or introducing bias concerning the meaning of the data. Whenever possible, research and sampling methods of the primary reports should be reported for each discrete item of data. When they cannot be reported due to brevity concerns, a description of the type of methodology used by the primary data sources should be mentioned. Results can then be reported as estimates of the total population sampled. Lastly, care should be taken that primary studies, which are published and hosted by governmental bodies as well as professional organizations, have followed approved **informed consent** procedures, and reporting of secondary data does not violate confidentiality of the original data sources or subjects. Informed consent is the voluntary agreement to participate in a study by individuals or agencies after they have received a complete explanation of the purpose, procedures, and risks and gains involved, and have understood the explanation.

Geographic Information Systems

Geographic information systems (GIS) use technology to maximize limited resources in identifying health and wellness needs in specific areas (Maguire, Goodchild, & Rhind, 1991). First developed in the 1960s, GIS is used by local and national governments in health and wellness assessment as well as in environmental planning and resource conservation (Stern, 1995). GIS uses a computerized program that includes hardware and software for identifying, locating, storing, integrating, mapping, analyzing, and illustrating data related to geographical locations locally and worldwide. Data can also be layered to create a richly detailed mapping of areas of need as well as areas of strength and current services provided. All data that it uses is geocoded to locate it accurately in any census block, and then analyzed using spatial analysis methods to produce a cost-effective mapping of public health data (Richards, Croner, Rushton, Brown, & Fowler, 1999). GIS is universally recognized as a powerful method of identifying, planning for, and predicting health and wellness needs.

HEALTHY PEOPLE 2010 GOALS AND OBJECTIVES FOR IMPROVING HEALTH

Healthy People was born in 1979 as *Healthy People: The Surgeon General's Report on Health Promotion and Disease Prevention* (U.S. Office of the Assistant Secretary for Health and Surgeon General, 1979). Its five goals aimed to reduce mortality rates among infants, children, adolescents, young adults, and older adults and to increase the independence of older adults. These goals were supported by objectives that were designed to operationalize the goals and drive interventions. **Objectives** are developed from and support the general goal. They are more specifically worded goals that can be measured over a specified period of time to evaluate the progress of the plan. The 467 objectives of *Healthy People 2010* are all designed to support its 28 goals. The first *Healthy People* document was followed in 1990 by *Healthy People 2000*, a national initiative to improve the general health of all people in the nation. *Healthy People 2000* consisted of three national health goals and 22 priority areas, supported by 319 health promotion and prevention objectives (U.S. Department of Health and Human Services, 1990).

Healthy People 2010 (U.S. Department of Health and Human Services, 2000) represents the third time that the DHHS has developed 10-year disease prevention and health promotion objectives for the nation. *Healthy People 2010* contains 467 objectives in 28 focus areas, or goals. Its **Leading Health Indicators** are measures used to predict future trends.

TABLE 1-2 Health Needs Assessment Process Methods

TYPE	DESCRIPTION	USE IN NEEDS ASSESSMENT
Focus Groups	Interviews with small, homogeneous group of individuals, usually community members, using open-ended questions.	Determine the expressed and felt needs and wants of members of a specific community. Provides qualitative insights that can't be derived from written questionnaires.
Key Informant Interviews	Interview with individuals recognized as having specific experience or expertise. Semistructured interview questionnaire or outline guides questions and encourages informants to share personal perspectives. Key informant is asked to recommend other key informants. Snowball sampling technique begins.	Can provide information and insights into the needs of a community or a specific group in a community. Allows interviewer to maximize the number of information-rich key informants over a short period of time.
Traditional Survey	Gathers data from a small sample that is representative of a larger population. Uses interview schedule, or outline of questions. Can be done by phone, Internet, mail, or personal interview.	Can be used to study any population. Determines expressed, normative, felt, and comparative needs of specific population groups.
Secondary Analysis of Existing Data	Identifying, gathering, grouping, and analyzing existing data from valid sources.	Focus groups and key informant interviews describe, illustrate, validate, and enrich data gathered from existing data. Especially useful for comparing sample characteristics.

continues

TABLE 1-2 Health Needs Assessment Process Methods *continued*

TYPE	DESCRIPTION	USE IN NEEDS ASSESSMENT
		Also useful when time and financial resources are limited
Geometric Information Systems (GIS)	Uses computerized program for identifying, locating, storing, integrating, mapping, analyzing, and illustrating data related to geographical locations worldwide	Technology provides best use of limited resources. Maps large areas. Data can be layered to provide rich descriptions of needs and resources.

They can provide baseline data on health behaviors to help individuals and communities target actions to improve health and achieve two overarching goals:

◆ Increase quality and years of healthy life

◆ Eliminate health disparities

The ten 2010 Leading Health Indicators are summarized in Box 1-3 and explained in depth in the following sections.

Physical Activity

An active lifestyle, which includes regular exercise, can contribute to the overall health and wellness of individuals and families. However, women are less active than men, and African Americans, Hispanics, and people with disabilities are less active than other population groups (Centers for Disease Control, 1998). The *Healthy People 2010* physical activity objectives aim to increase the number of adolescents and adults who engage in physical activity on a regular basis, as well as the time involved in such activity (U.S. Department of Health and Human Services, 2000).

Overweight and Obesity

Obesity and weight problems contribute to health problems, especially diabetes, cardiovascular and respiratory conditions, chronic joint and back pain, and certain types of cancers. The social and personal costs of obesity include lower economic status, low self-esteem, and discrimination (National Institutes of Health, 1998). The *Healthy People 2010* overweight and obesity objectives aim to reduce the proportion of adults, children and adolescents who are overweight or obese (U.S. Department of Health and Human Services, 2000).

Tobacco Use

Cigarette smoking accounts for more preventable deaths than drug and alcohol use and abuse, motor vehicle accidents, suicide, firearms, suicide, and AIDS combined. Yet more than one-third of adolescents smoke, and this number is steadily increasing. Exposure to tobacco and its smoke before and after birth is implicated in miscarriage, sudden infant death syndrome, and childhood asthma and bronchitis (Centers for Disease Control, 1997). The *Healthy People 2010* tobacco use objectives target the reduction of tobacco use by adolescents and adults (U.S. Department of Health and Human Services, 2000).

> **Box 1-3 ▪ The Ten HP 2010 Leading Health Indicators***
>
> 1. *Physical Activity*
> 2. *Overweight and Obesity*
> 3. *Tobacco Use*
> 4. *Substance Abuse*
> 5. *Responsible Sexual Behavior*
> 6. *Mental Health*
> 7. *Injury and Violence*
> 8. *Environmental quality*
> 9. *Immunizations*
> 10. *Access to Health Care*
>
> * *U.S. Department of Health and Human Services. (January, 2000).* Healthy people 2010. *(Conference Edition, in Volume I).Washington, DC., p. 24.*

Substance Abuse

The use of illegal psychoactive substances and the abuse of prescription medications and alcohol is a leading health indicator. It is associated with a number of chronic health conditions, such as cirrhosis of the liver, communicable diseases such as HIV infection, infant developmental disorders such as fetal alcohol syndrome, accidents involving firearms and motor vehicles, family and individual abuse, and community violence (Bullock & Henze, 2000; SAMHSA, 1999). *Healthy People 2010* goals seek to increase the proportion of adults and adolescents who do not use alcohol or any illicit substances or engage in any binge drinking in any given month (U.S. Department of Health and Human Services, 2000).

Responsible Sexual Behavior

Unsafe sexual behaviors can be defined as acts not protected by use of a barrier, by pregnancy pre-planning, or through a safe mutual adult relationship. Unintended and adolescent pregnancies, sexually transmitted diseases, HIV infections, and AIDS pose costs to society in terms of loss of quality of life and rates of illness (American Social Health Association, 1998; Maynard, 1997) *Healthy People 2010* goals aim to increase rates of abstinence for adolescents or increase the rates of condom use among those adolescents and adults who are sexually active (U.S. Department of Health and Human Services, 2000).

Mental Health

Clinical depression and other mood disorders remain the most prevalent form of mental illness in the United States (Mayberg, Mahurin, & Brannon, 1997). Mental disorders create an economic burden on individuals, families, and society in the forms of stress and suffering, loss of quality of life, jobs, and participation in relationships, family life, and community endeavors (Greenberg, 1993). *Healthy People 2010* goals seek to improve prompt identification and effective treatment of mood disorders and mental illness (U.S. Department of Health and Human Services, 2000).

Injury and Violence

Our violent society is the troubling context in which babies are born and grow, children are schooled and play, adults couple and raise families, and communities are built and attempt to prosper. Society as a whole is concerned about impaired driving from the use of drugs or alcohol and gunshot wounds and homicides, particularly among African Americans, who are murdered at a much higher rate than Whites (Hoyert, Kochanek, & Murphy, 1999). *Healthy People 2010* goals are aimed at reducing intentional and unintentional injuries, particularly those due to motor vehicle accidents and homicides (U.S. Department of Health and Human Services, 2000).

Environmental

In our global society, the environment is everyone's concern. As our increasingly mobile societies cross national borders, they can bring with them previously contained infectious diseases and biologic and chemical hazards. Environmental hazards such as secondhand smoke, poor sanitation, damage to the ozone layer, air pollution and poor air quality, polluted water and waterways, vector-borne diseases, and biological and chemical pollution contribute to at least 25 percent of preventable illnesses globally (WHO Information Fact Sheets, 1997). *Healthy People 2010* goals seek to reduce the rate of exposure to secondhand smoke and other environmental hazards (U.S. Department of Health and Human Services, 2000).

Immunization

Childhood immunization rates are over 90 percent for the recommended vaccinations such as smallpox, polio, and measles (Centers for Disease Control and Prevention, 1998). For adults, immunization rates for pneumococcal pneumonia and influenza are significantly lower for African Americans and Hispanics than for Whites. Less than half of older adults who are at risk for medical complications or death from influenza receive vaccinations against the disease (Prevention and Control of Influenza, April 14, 2000). *Healthy People 2010* goals aim to increase the immunization rate for recommended vaccines for children under five as well as for adults and the elderly (U.S. Department of Health and Human Services, 2000).

Access to Health Care

Access to quality health care is influenced by insurance coverage, having an ongoing relationship with a primary health care provider, and socioeconomic status. A significant number of adults and families with young children are without health insurance (Centers for Disease Control and Prevention, 1995). Language barriers, cultural practices and beliefs, and lack of transportation can also limit access to primary health care services and prenatal health care in the first trimester of pregnancy. *Healthy People 2010* goals focus on increasing the number of individuals and families with health insurance, increasing the number who have an ongoing source of primary health care, and increasing the number of pregnant women who receive prenatal care in the first trimester of pregnancy (U.S. Department of Health and Human Services, 2000).

Goals, Objectives, and Benchmarks

The general *Healthy People 2010* goals, as presented above, are broad statements that direct health assessment and intervention efforts. These general goals were then used to develop 28 health promotion and disease prevention focus areas. These 28 goals are listed in Box 1-4.

These goals provide direction for the development of objectives. Objectives, in turn, focus health prevention and promotion actions. The objectives use the **determinants of health** to promote health, prevent disease, and ensure access to quality health care. Determinants of health are critical influences, such as individual lifestyles, biologic makeup and behaviors, community physical and social environments, access to health care, and policies and health interventions that combine to determine the health and wellness of individuals, families, and communities (McGinnis & Malese, 1997; Syme & Balfour, 1998).

Benchmarks are targets for performance or outcomes that indicate a goal has been reached. The needs assessment model presented in this book uses the *Healthy People 2010* objectives and targeted outcomes as its benchmarks, and compares data to these benchmarks in order to determine the status of a community's health and wellness. The 28 *Healthy People 2010* goals will be described in more detail in subsequent chapters.

Box 1-4 ■ Healthy People 2010 Goals

1. *Access to quality health services*
2. *Arthritis, osteoporosis, and chronic back conditions*
3. *Cancer*
4. *Chronic kidney disease*
5. *Diabetes*
6. *Disability and secondary conditions*
7. *Educational and community-based programs*
8. *Environmental health*
9. *Family planning*
10. *Food safety*
11. *Health communication*
12. *Heart disease and stroke*
13. *HIV*
14. *Immunization and infectious diseases*
15. *Injury and violence prevention*
16. *Maternal, infant, and child health*
17. *Medical product safety*
18. *Mental health and mental disorders*
19. *Nutrition and overweight*
20. *Occupational safety and health*
21. *Oral health*
22. *Physical activity and fitness*
23. *Public health infrastructure*
24. *Respiratory diseases*
25. *Sexually transmitted diseases*
26. *Substance abuse*
27. *Tobacco use*
28. *Vision and hearing*

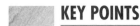 **KEY POINTS**

◆ The purpose of a health and wellness needs assessment can serve as a foundation for improved communication and cooperation within a community in identification of health and wellness service and evaluation needs.

◆ A needs assessment is a critical first step in determining the state of health and wellness in any community or in developing health and wellness programs or projects for a community or population group.

◆ The World Health Organization defines health as more than the absence of illness or disease; it is a state of complete wellness that incorporates social factors such as socioeconomic status, education, safety, and the environment.

◆ Theoretical models of community health and health needs assessment include the community-as-partner, ecological, health behavior, and health belief models.

◆ The Ontario Needs Impact Based Model is used to define and describe the needs assessment problem, determine what information is required, gather the data, and analyze that information, using a valid basis of comparison, such as the *Healthy People 2010* goals and objectives as benchmarks or targets for performance.

◆ The steps of a community needs assessment include definition and description of needs assessment problem; determining what information is required; information gathering; and analysis of selected data.

◆ Secondary analysis of existing data is a survey method that uses existing data to reanalyze a set of quantitative data by combining and integrating data from several existing databases to examine new research questions.

◆ Geographic Information Systems (GIS) is a computerized mapping of data that provides a richly detailed illustration of resources and needs that can be used for health and wellness needs identification, planning, and predicting.

◆ The 10 Leading Health Indicators that *Healthy People 2010* targets to improve health and wellness are: physical activity, overweight and obesity, tobacco use, substance abuse, responsible sexual behavior, mental health, injury and violence, environmental, immunizations, and access to health care.

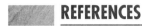 **REFERENCES**

Aday, L., & Anderson, R. (1974). A framework for the study of access to medical care. *Health Services Research, 9*, 208–220.

American Social Health Association. (1998). *Sexually transmitted diseases in America: How many cases and at what cost?* Menlo Park, CA: Kaiser Family Foundation.

Anderson, E., & McFarlane, J. (2000). *Community as partner* (4th ed.). Philadelphia: Lippincott.

Anderson, R., & Newman, J. (1973). Societal and individual determinants of medical care utilization in the United States. *Milbank Quarterly, 51*, 95–124.

Bronfenbrenner, U. (1979). Contexts of childrearing. *American Psychologist, 34*, 844–850.

Bullock, B., & Henze, R. (2000). *Focus on pathophysiology.* Philadelphia: Lippincott.

Centers for Disease Control and Prevention. (1995). Health insurance coverage and receipt of preventive health services—United States, 1993. *Morbidity and Mortality Weekly Report, 44* (11), 219–225.

Centers for Disease Control and Prevention. (1999). National vaccination coverage levels among children aged 19–35 months—United States, 1998. *Morbidity and Mortality Weekly Report, 48*, 829–830.

Centers for Disease Control and Prevention. (1999). Prevalence of sedentary leisure-time behaviors among adults in the United States. Health E-Stats. Atlanta: Centers of Disease Control and Prevention, National Center for Health Statistics.

Centers for Disease Control and Prevention (2000, April 14). Prevention and control of influenza: Recommendations of the Advisory Committee on Immunization Practices. *Morbidity and Mortality Weekly Report, 49*, (RR-3).

Centers for Disease Control and Prevention. (1997). Youth Risk Behavior Surveillance—United States. *Morbidity and Mortality Weekly Report, 47* (SS-3).

Garbarino, J. (1990). The human ecology of early risk. In S. Meisels & J. Shonkoff (Eds.), *Handbook of early childhood intervention* (pp. 78–96). Cambridge, MA: Cambridge University Press.

Graves, J. (1998). Secondary data analysis. In J. Fitzpatrick (Ed.), *Encyclopedia of nursing research* (pp. 523–524). New York: Springer.

Greenberg, P. (1993). The economic burden of depression in 1990. *Journal of Clinical Psychiatry, 54*, 405–418.

Heale, J., & Abernathy, T. (1996). Community health planning: Determining the needs of the community [online]. Available: http://cwhweb.mdmaster.ca/planning/itch96.htm.

Heale, J., Webster, G., & Abernathy, T. (1996, January.). *Community health planning: Determining the needs of the community.* Paper presented at the meeting of ITCH: A conference addressing information technology issues in community health. Victoria, BC.

Hothersall, D. (1995). *History of psychology.* New York: McGraw-Hill.

Hoyert, D., Kochanek, K., & Murphy, S. (1999). *Deaths: Final data for 1997.*

National Vital Statistics Reports, 47 (19). Hyattsville, MD: National Center for Health Statistics.

Huq, S. (1999). An interview with Dr. Pamela Hartigan. Health Promotion: *Global Perspectives, 2 (3),* 4–7.

Kerlinger, F., & Lee, H. (2000). *Foundations of behavioral research.* New York: Harcourt College.

Jane, N., & Becker, M. (1984). The health belief model: A decade later. *Health Education Quarterly, 11,* 1–47.

Maguire, D., Goodchild, M., & Rhind, D. (1991). *Geographical information systems: Principles and applications.* New York: Longman.

Mayberg, H., Mahurin, R., & Brannon, S. (1997). Neuropsychiatric aspects of mood disorder and affective disorders. In S. Yudofsky & R. Hales (Eds.), *The American Psychiatric Press textbook of neuropsychiatry* (3rd ed.), pp. 883–902.Washington, DC: American Psychiatric Press.

Maynard, R. (1997). *Kids having kids: Economic costs and social consequences of teen pregnancy.* Washington, DC: Urban Institute Press.

McGinnis, J., & Malese, D. (1997). Defining mission, goals and objectives. In F. Scutchfield & C. Keck (Eds.), *Principles of public health practice* (pp. 136–145). Clifton Park, NY: Delmar Learning.

National Institutes of Health. (1998, February 12). *Statistics related to overweight and obesity.* NIH Publication no. 96-4158. National Institute of Diabetes and Digestive and Kidney Diseases. Bethesda, MD: U.S. Department of Health.

Nieswiadomy, R. (2002). *Foundations of nursing research.* Upper Saddle River, NJ: Prentice Hall.

O'Brien, R. (1998). An overview of the methodological approach of action research. Action research methodology. Available: http://www.web.net/~robrien/papers/arfinal.html.

Patton, M. (1990). *Qualitative evaluation and research methods.* Newbury Park, CA: Sage.

Perry, C.,Williams, C., Mortenson, S., Toomey, T., Komro, K., Anstime, P., McGovern, P., Finnegan, J., Forster, J., Wagenaar, A., & Wolfson, M. (1996). Project Northland: Outcomes of a community-wide alcohol use prevention program during adolescence. *American Journal of Public Health, 86,* 956–965.

Polit, D., & Hungler, B. (1997). Essentials of nursing research: *Methods, appraisals and utilization* (4th ed.). Philadelphia: Lippincott.

Prevention and Control of Influenza. Recommendations of the Advisory Committee on Immunization Practices (ACIP) (April 14, 2000). *Morbidity and Mortality Weekly Report.*

Richards, T., Croner, C., Rushton, G., Brown, C., & Fowler, L. (1999). Geographic information systems and public health: Mapping the future. *Public Health Reports, 114,* 359–373.

Rosenstock, I. (1990). The Health Belief Model: Explaining health behavior through expectancies. In K. Glanz, F. Lewis, & B. Rimer (Eds.), *Health behavior and education* (pp. 39–63). San Francisco: Jossey-Bass.

SAMSHSA. (1999). Summary of findings from the 1998 National Household Survey on Drug Abuse. Rockville, MD: HHS, SAMHSA, Office of Applied Studies.

Schutt, R. (2001). *Investigating the social world* (3rd ed.). Boston: Pine Forge.

Shellman, J. (2000, July/August). Promoting elder wellness through a community-based blood pressure clinic. *Public Health Nursing, 17,* 257–263.

Stern, R. (1995). The added value of Geographical Information Systems in public and environmental health. In R. Stern (Ed.), *Environmental and health data in Europe as a tool for risk management: Needs, uses and strategies* (pp. 3–24). Hingham, MA: Kluwer Academic.

Stokols, D. (1992). Establishing and maintaining healthy environments: Toward a social ecology of health promotion. *American Psychologist. 47,* 6–22.

Syme, S., & Balfour, J. (1998). *Social determinants of disease.* In R. Wallace (Ed.), *Public health and preventive medicine* (14th ed., p. 795). Stamford, CT: Appleton & Lange.

Trachim, W. (2000). *The research methods knowledge base.* Cincinnati, OH: Atomic Dog Publishers, Hybrid Media.

U.S. Department of Health and Human Services. (1990). *Healthy People 2000: National health promotion and disease prevention objectives.* Washington, DC: U.S. Government Printing Office.

U.S. Department of Health and Human Services. (2000, January). *Healthy People 2010* (Conference Edition, in Two Volumes). Washington, DC.

U.S. Office of the Assistant Secretary for Health and Surgeon General. (1979). *Healthy People: The surgeon general's report on health promotion and disease prevention.* Washington DC: U.S. Government Printing Office.

Wilson, H. (1993). *Introducing research in nursing* (2nd ed.). Redwood City, CA: Addison-Wesley Nursing.

World Health Organization. (1946). Constitution of the World Health Organization. *American Journal of Public Health, 36,* 1315–1323.

World Health Organization. (1986). Health and welfare Canada and Canadian Public Health Association. *Ottawa Charter for Health Promotion.* Copenhagen: World Health Organization.

World Health Organization. (2001). Definition of health. *About WHO.* Available: www.who.int/aboutwho/en/definition.html.

WHO Information Fact Sheets. (1997, June). *Health and Environment in sustainable development.* Fact Sheet No. 170. Geneva: World Health Organization.

2

STEPS OF THE COMMUNITY HEALTH AND WELLNESS NEEDS ASSESSMENT PROCESS

Deena A. Nardi

LEARNING OBJECTIVES

At the conclusion of this chapter, the reader will be able to:

- ◆ Obtain informed consent before beginning a needs assessment.
- ◆ Define and describe a needs assessment problem.
- ◆ Form a community coalition for the purpose of conducting a needs assessment.
- ◆ Identify pertinent information required for assessment.
- ◆ Compare the indicators assessed to *Healthy People 2010* benchmarks.
- ◆ Construct a needs assessment tool.

KEY TERMS

Coalition

Comparative needs

Conceptual framework

Developmental goal

Epidemiological study

Expressed needs

Felt needs

Informed consent

Key informants

Normative needs

Primary health care

T his chapter discusses the steps of the needs assessment process in further detail, beginning with the need to address confidentiality of data and issues of informed consent. This chapter also illustrates the process, application, and credibility of secondary analysis of existing documents as one method of needs assessment that is rigorous, cost-effective, and useful in action research studies throughout the nation. A completed needs assessment tool demonstrates how identified data can be compared with benchmarks to determine the current health and wellness status and current health systems operations of a selected community, using a tricounty area as a representational sampling. This practice model provides a tool for use by nurse educators, the academic community, and public health and service operations to assist in addressing regional health and wellness outcomes.

BEFORE BEGINNING: INFORMED CONSENT

All health and human services providers, from nurses, physicians, and social workers to teachers and therapists, subscribe to a professional code of ethics unique to their professions. These codes of ethics identify the general rights and responsibilities of members of that profession regarding the protection of the public and the preservation of that public's rights (Burkhardt & Nathaniel, 1998). The ethical code for nurses, which specifically identifies the nurses' responsibility to safeguard the client's rights to privacy and confidentiality, is contained in the American Nurses Association *Code for Nurses* (1997). The ethical principles that guide physician practice also counsel physicians to deal honestly with and safeguard their clients' confidentiality within the constraints of the law (American Medical Association, 2000).

Ethical codes require that any population to be directly surveyed or measured must freely consent to participate in the study prior to beginning a needs assessment (Sultz & Young, 1999). **Informed consent** is designed to protect people and institutions from any harm, experimentation, or exploitation. It is the voluntary agreement to participate in a study by individuals or agencies after they have received a complete explanation of the purpose, procedures, and risks and gains involved, and have understood the explanation. To obtain informed consent, the purpose, procedures used, nature of the person's participation, all possible risks and known benefits must be explained to each subject, and then measures must be taken to determine that the subject has understood the explanation and freely consents to the assessment (Patton, 1990; Cherry & Jacob, 1999). Care must be taken, therefore, to tailor any explanation to the learning and developmental level and circumstances of the subject.

Obtaining informed consent cannot be accomplished in the traditional manner when conducting a needs assessment using secondary analysis of existing data, since the data is available to all as public records (Schutt, 2001). However, the assessment team still has the responsibility of determining if all secondary data was gathered by the primary researchers using proper research techniques, such as their having obtained approval by the human subjects review committee associated with the study, and by their having secured informed consent. This kind of information is archived with the original data set in the public records, along with such information as study purpose and method, operational definitions, and sampling criteria.

Once informed consent is obtained, the four steps of the needs assessment process can begin.

STEP ONE: DEFINITION AND DESCRIPTION OF THE PROBLEM

Any group or individual can design, develop, and implement a needs assessment regardless of the resources and funding available to them, if the participants are invested in the work, if the plan is clearly mapped out, and if strategies are in place for obtaining and evaluating results. The first step of the community health and wellness needs assessment is to decide why and where the assessment should be done. In other words, explain the problem, identify where it is occurring or where it might occur by designating the area or group you wish to survey, and then describe your purpose. For example, the purpose of the needs assessment might be to secure external funds to support a health or wellness program in a community, to evaluate access to health services for a specific population group (e.g., perhaps you are concerned about what percentage of pregnant women in a city or rural area receive prenatal care during their first trimester of pregnancy), or to determine the current health or wellness status for a particular location, such as a neighborhood, a community, a township, or a city.

The purpose is identified by posing a question concerning health or wellness, which might arise from personal or professional experience (Schutt, 2001). For instance, a nurse practitioner (NP) might note that victims of assault who were treated at one hospital were always visited by a rape/assault counselor prior to their hospital discharge. He or she might wonder if the pre-discharge counseling visit is standard practice in all city or regional hospitals, or if practices vary from hospital to hospital. The health assessment question arising from this observation might be, "Do all hospitals provide sexual assault counseling before discharge?" This question would need to be refined to a measurable and manageable size. After discussing the observation and initial question with colleagues, the more refined health assessment question developed to start the assessment process might be, "What are the policies, procedures and practices for treatment of a victim of sexual assault in all hospitals in this city?" This question frames the inquiry, and also leads to further questions related to this original health assessment question, which will in turn provide needed data that more accurately presents the results. The question calls for a survey of policies, a list of treatment actions and resources (procedures), and a time line of treatment steps taken from arrival at the hospital emergency room until discharge from hospital treatment (who does what to whom and when).

The purpose of the survey would be to determine if it is standard practice for adults in one specified city to receive counseling from a qualified source before they left a city hospital. Results might be used for the development of a citywide counseling program for all victims of sexual assault regardless of which hospital treated and released them. On the other hand, results might show that all city hospitals provided some type of counseling prior to discharge for any adult assault victims, and such a program is not needed. Or results might show that this supportive service was available to all women, but not routinely available to men. So the need in that case would be to design and implement a citywide counseling program for adult male victims of sexual assault.

In the example presented below and used throughout this text, an excerpt of one health and well-being needs assessment is provided that illustrates how the assessment team has identified their purpose and then used it to guide their first step of the assessment process:

A group of educators and community leaders in one Midwest region decided to assess the region's health and well-being needs in order to better understand them and their implications for **primary health care** and human services program development. Primary health care is the point of health care service where consumers first enter the health care system. For child-bearing women, this might be the obstetrician/gynecologist; for a young child, primary health care would first begin with the pediatrician or pediatric nurse practitioner. Primary health care is different from primary prevention, which describes the prevention of illness in a population through such activities as wellness assessment and education (U.S. Preventative Services Task Force, 1996).

The resulting regional health and well-being needs assessment would serve as a foundation for improved community communication and cooperation in identification of health and well-being service and evaluation needs. It could also stimulate a greater collaboration among campus and community health care providers, community groups, institutions, and organizations. The needs identified in the report could serve to provide direction to county Education and Health Departments as they prioritized and deployed their resources.

The purpose of the team's health and wellness needs assessment was to provide comprehensive documentation of the current health and well-being status and current health systems operations of a Midwestern region, using a tricounty area as a representational sampling. This proposed **epidemiological study** would be used to develop externally funded projects that advanced community health and well-being. An epidemiological study is a type of action research that examines the distribution and determinants of health and wellness-related states for identified populations. The first step toward that goal, a health and wellness needs assessment, would be conducted by a multidisciplinary team of health and human services providers, including physicians, nurses, teachers, social workers, community leaders, and university students (Nardi, Sutherland, Tippy & Strupeck, 2000).

Creating community investment in the health and wellness needs assessment is key to its success in gathering relevant data and implementing any recommendations that derive from its conclusions (Wandersman, Goodman, & Butterfoss, 1997). A team comprised of individuals who are cooperating to conduct a needs assessment can accomplish this task more effectively than one person working alone. The team can provide a broader perspective, more resources, a wider variety of skills, and a stronger decision-making process than can be achieved by a person working alone. The key to effective teamwork is the formation of a **coalition,** or a group of individuals who are key representatives of the community who are partnering, sharing resources, and cooperating to achieve the same goals (Aspen Reference Group, 1997). In this case, the goal is to produce an accurate health and wellness needs assessment. Coalitions are a necessary component of any community health and wellness assessment, since all community health endeavors should be conducted in partnership with the community.

The steps of coalition building as described above can be grouped into four major activities:

1. Defining goals and objectives
2. Identifying the problem
3. Engaging community leaders or interested parties who would want to be involved
4. Maintaining the coalition

Defining Goals and Objectives

The first step is deciding what you want to accomplish. In the example of community health and wellness needs assessment that is presented throughout this book, the coalition first discussed the individual concerns that brought them to first meet. They then agreed on what they could accomplish that would benefit them collectively and individually as special interest representatives. Due to a narrow time frame and limited resources, they decided that they would assess the community health and wellness needs of three large counties in one region of their Midwestern state instead of trying to do a regionwide assessment. This agreement enabled them to focus their activities and maximize their resources. In the other example provided, the NP defined the objective of the assessment as determining if all hospitalized adult victims of sexual assault received counseling prior to discharge.

Identifying the Problem

The problem statement can be first developed in the form of an assessment question, as already described. Then, *Healthy People 2010* goals and objectives assist in framing the problem in terms of location, demographics (age, gender, socioeconomic status) of the population involved, and expected results. In one of the examples offered previously, the NP identifies the problem as not knowing if all adult victims of sexual assault received counseling prior to hospital discharge. The expected results would be that all victims receive appropriate counseling prior to hospital discharge after assault, which addresses the *Healthy People 2010* goal 18: "Improve mental health and ensure access to appropriate, quality mental health services" (U.S. Department of Health and Human Services, 2000, p. 18–3).

Engaging Community Leaders or Interested Parties Who Would Want to Be Involved

Consider the assets that key members of the community who might not be connected to the health care industry might bring to the coalition. Small business owners, educators, family caretakers, and lawyers, for example, can bring personal experience and resources to the coalition to help it obtain its goals. In the example of the regional community assessment coalition, the team included a lawyer, an accountant, a politician, several teachers, some community activists, a physicist, and several advanced practice nurses. They received a written invitation to join the coalition, followed by several follow-up calls by the coalition chair. At their first meeting, the chair asked the group what they hoped to accomplish. Their responses were then linked to develop the overall goal of the coalition, which was to document the current health and wellness status and current health systems operations of their region, as a step to develop externally funded projects that advanced health and wellness in their communities.

In the other example given, the NP might want to meet with the director of nurses or hospital CEOs to explain the purpose of the proposed needs assessment, how it might be conducted, and the benefit this needs assessment can provide to the hospital. In the example given previously, hospitals can use the results of the assessment to determine how well they are doing in reaching the *Healthy People 2010* objective 18–6: "Increase the number of persons seen in primary health care who receive mental health screening and assessment" (U.S. Department of Health and Human Services, 2000, p. 18–16). Explaining how key players or community leaders can benefit from the assessment engages them in the project, and produces team members who are personally invested in joining the coalition.

Maintaining the Coalition

The coalition needs nurturing, refreshing, and strengthening to enable individual members with diverse priorities and perspectives to remain focused on the task at hand (to develop, conduct, and use a health and wellness needs assessment). To keep the coalition fresh and functioning, the assessment team leader should take a number of steps:

◆ Know the coalition members and be familiar with their goals. Ask them about their individual and collective goals, what they would like to see happen for themselves, their families, and their communities. Only by doing this and showing genuine interest in their concerns can a team leader keep the diverse members of a collaborative effort engaged in a collective task.

◆ Keep meetings short and to the point. Develop and stick to an agenda for the meeting. Try to set a one-hour time frame for each meeting. When meetings are long, they can discourage attendance, and missing meetings is the first step toward an individual's disengagement. The adage "less is more" can be applied to time frame as well as choice of meeting topics. Information can be outlined and presented as handouts that committee members can take with them to study at a more convenient time. Keeping the meetings short and to the point communicates that you value the committee members' time and attendance, and that you will not take advantage of it.

◆ Stay in touch with members, sending them timely reminders of all meetings and activities. Leave phone messages as well as send notes or memos before each meeting. Determine if the meeting place is accessible to all members and accommodates persons with disabilities. Phone members who miss a meeting. Assure them that their contribution is valued, and inquire about how you can help them make the next meeting.

◆ Begin each meeting with a list of what is to be accomplished during the meeting, and end the meeting with a summary of what was accomplished. This summary provides a sense that the committee is moving forward in accomplishing its goals, that the goals will be met, and that their time has been well spent.

Becoming familiar with the individual goals of the coalition members is a central task role of the coalition chair(s). Coalition members come to the table with diverse backgrounds and interests, and with other role responsibilities, obligations, and demands on their time. If they do not see a clear connection between their participation as coalition members and the goals and accomplishments of the coalition, the coalition's assessment activities will cease to be a priority, and they will stop contributing or cease coming to meetings altogether. The chair should know what members want to accomplish, and then articulate how the assessment activities can contribute to members' individual goals.

STEP TWO: DETERMINING WHAT INFORMATION IS REQUIRED

The *Healthy People 2010* focus areas for improving the health of the nation are used in this model as a **conceptual framework**, or road map (Chitty, 2001), for choosing the areas of health and wellness related to concerns that should be assessed and the information required to do so. A conceptual framework is a theory about a group of constructs that are systematically organized and related in some way for a purpose. The idea lends a focus for examining and understanding the concepts, and gathering and interpreting information concerning the concepts. A conceptual framework can evolve from the experiences and intuitive insights of experts in a field, and represents a certain way of thinking about a situation or phenomenon. *Healthy People 2010,* for instance, presents an umbrella of goals for improving the health of the nation that systematically organizes the data and concerns of a multitude of government, public, and private health organizations in the United States into 28 focus areas.

These focus areas, termed goals by *Healthy People 2010,* now provide one organizing framework for diverse people and organizations to help define and locate data concerning health and wellness in areas of particular concern to them, using these goals and objectives as **normative needs.** Normative needs are the benchmarks described by *Healthy People 2010.* They are recognized standards for health outcomes for population groups in the aggregate. They were developed by a large coalition of experts and key informants in health and human services under the auspices of the U.S. Department of Health and Humans Services (U.S. Department of Health and Human Services, 2000). Each of the 28 goals are supported and further defined by a number of objectives that serve to operationalize the goals.

In the example provided in this chapter, the NP and the assessment team would review all focus areas and then identify the goal that appears to relate to their first question: "Do all hospitals provide sexual assault counseling before discharge?" This goal would be goal 18: "Improve mental health and ensure access to appropriate, quality mental health services" (U.S. Department of Health and Human Services, 2000, p. 18–3). The objective under this goal that would most clearly operationalize this goal would be objective 18–6, "Increase the number of persons seen in primary health care who receive mental health screening and assessment" (U.S. Department of Health and Human Services, 2000, p. 18–16).

Primary health care refers to the point at which a client enters the health care system, and includes emergency room services, HMOs, health clinics, work sites, and health care provider offices (Aydelotte, 1983;

Lundy & Janes, 2001). In the United States, the uninsured and underinsured customarily use the emergency room as their primary health care provider (Frisch & Frisch, 2002), because they believe that they will not be turned away for lack of insurance and they have no other regular primary health care provider. Because of this situation, it is essential for the assessment team to use strategies to include the homeless, uninsured, and underinsured when gathering data about primary health care needs and use.

Chapters 3 to 7 present strategies for locating data from these hidden populations in needs assessments. In the example given above, the place in which the victim of sexual assault would first receive health care services would most probably be the emergency room. The sexual assault counseling services received there would include screening and assessment for rape-trauma-related mental health disorders or concerns. The objective mentioned above speaks to the need for health care providers to provide a visit by a counselor trained in sexual assault and rape trauma counseling, who will screen and assess for further need of mental health services. Because this goal is presented as a **developmental goal,** there are no target data to benchmark for comparison. A developmental goal is established whenever there is a need to develop a baseline of information about the phenomenon under study. So the NP and assessment team will choose to survey all hospital emergency rooms in their city to determine how many offer pre-discharge counseling services. The secondary question, "What are the policies, procedures, and practices for treatment of a victim of sexual assault in all hospitals in this city?" serves to identify the information the assessment team needs to gather.

STEP THREE: INFORMATION GATHERING

The goal of information gathering is to obtain useful data about the community and its health and wellness needs (Lundy & Janes, 2001). Assessment teams use many different sources to gather data. Primary sources include the key informants in the community who can offer accurate insights and current understandings based on their experiences with the subject. Key informants are the political, business, health, and spiritual leaders in the community, as well as consumers who are directly affected by health issues addressed in the problem statement or question (Allender & Spradley, 2001). In the example used in this chapter, the assessment team would contact hospital emergency room administrators to explain the need for and purpose of the assessment and arrange to interview them concerning written policies and procedures for sexual assault victim counseling prior to hospital discharge.

If the assessment team is using secondary analysis of existing data and analysis of public records as the method of identifying and gathering existing data, then valid sources must be first identified. There are many types of valid sources readily available to the assessment team, including published reports on the identified goal or objective; state and local census data; existing needs assessments or reports; key informants in the region; community groups; informed consumers; and other local or federal databases on the Internet, by request or through the library (Rodeghier, 1996). The web is recognized as an excellent place to gather data from neighborhood, city, county, state, and federal sources. (Chapter 8 provides a cross-referenced list of currently available national, state, and regional resources that can be useful in gathering data pertinent to community health issues.) Again, using the example above, after interviewing the emergency room administrators and obtaining their permission, the assessment team would collect copies of the written policies and procedures concerning sexual assault victim counseling prior to hospital discharge from each hospital source, in order to determine if policies routinely existed and what they consist of.

Primary and secondary data provide a baseline of information that can be used to compare with *Healthy People 2010* objectives and targeted outcomes when determining **comparative needs.** Comparative needs are the identified determinants of health as identified by *Healthy People 2010* for a specific population, which are compared to the health behaviors outcome data for a specific population.

These comparative needs can be validated through individual or group interviews with key informants, as well as through questionnaires and anecdotal reporting by key informants to identify **expressed needs.** Expressed needs related to health are the needs that are already identified by the users and providers of health care and community services in a community.

Small groups of informed consumers as well as other key informants will also discuss their **felt needs**, which can inform and validate the existing data the team is also collecting through secondary means. Felt needs are expressed needs that are subjectively experienced by a person or population. They are experienced personally as being lacking or desired. A felt need may be shaped by a person's perceptions of the desirability of achieving a health indicator, or accessibility to services.

Other sources of secondary data include international sources, such as the World Health Organization and its six regional offices, other health organizations, and the World Federation of Public Health Associations, all accessible on the Internet. National or federal resources include the data banks that are available on the Internet or can be purchased through the mail. These agencies include the American Public Health Association, the National Institute for Health, the U.S. Public Health Service (USPHS), the U.S. Bureau of the Census, the Agency for Healthcare Research and Quality, and the U.S. Department of Health and Human Services. Internet addresses for these agencies and others are provided in Chapter 8.

Community and regional sources can be located by first using a snowball sampling method of obtaining information (Schutt, 1999). In snowball sampling, a **key informant** is asked where to obtain specific health assessment information that her or his organization might have collected or is included in reports. A key informant is an information-rich provider and user of health care services who is recognized as having experience or expertise with a specific issue, and who can provide valuable information and insights into the needs of a community or a specific group within the community.

The key informant might refer to other community sources for further data. The key informant would also be asked if she or he knew of any other sources for current data that addresses the *Healthy People 2010* objective and its target benchmark. The key informant would mention other sources, and these sources would be approached and queried, thus widening the range of sources for community and regional data that can be reached for secondary analysis of existing data. Many state and community agencies have their own data banks containing population demographics that they maintain on specific health issues they are interested in. Many of these data banks are available to the consumer on the Internet or by contacting the state chapter or headquarters of agency.

STEP FOUR: ANALYSIS OF THE INFORMATION

In any health and wellness needs assessment, the analysis of the data requires an integrated and unified interpretation of the data (Strauss, 2000). This interpretive process requires several steps. Chapter 7 provides a detailed explanation of these steps of the analysis process. The steps are presented here in summary form to provide a general overview of the analysis process.

The first step in analyzing the information collected is to reexamine the data. It should be examined for any omissions, mislabeling, or errors before entering it into an electronic file for storage and categorization for later analysis. Also, anything unusual or unexpected about the data should be rechecked for accuracy before proceeding. This can easily be accomplished by verifying the data through tracing its source, then rechecking for transcription or omission errors (Rodeghier, 1996).

The data is then categorized according to the model of health assessment you choose to use. The 28 goals of *Healthy People 2010* are used in this text to categorize health and wellness needs because of their compatibility with the Ontario Needs Impact Based Model of health and wellness needs assessment, and the use of a secondary analysis of existing data methodology.

The data is then compared with the *Healthy People 2010* objectives and target benchmarks for similar populations and areas for congruency of terms and population as well as results. For instance, in the example provided below, one assessment team uses the objective 1–2, "Increase the proportion of persons who have a specific source of ongoing care" (U.S. Department of Health and Human Services, 2000, p. 1–14), to guide their search for information about access to health care for the population in their region. Using the latest community health assessment report published by a major city in their region, they discover that 13.5 percent of area adults do not seek medical care because of the cost, compared to 7.0 percent of U.S. adults, and that area parents are twice as apt as parents in the whole United States not to seek medical care for their children because of the cost.

This comparison is then used to form logical conclusions about the data and whether it indicates the existence of a health and well-being need. This process of forming logical conclusions is also called drawing inferences from the data (Anderson & McFarlane, 2000). Cultural differences and socioeconomic levels as well as education levels and language usage must be considered when drawing inferences. The inferences that are developed are then summarized, and this information is then included in a final summary of results. Table 2-1 presents a brief acronym for remembering and applying this four-step process model.

An example of how one health assessment team formed inferences from the data comparison, and then summarized them to identify health and well-being needs, is presented below. In this example, the summary addresses the diversity of the region as well as the hidden uninsured working poor as it identifies its regional needs:

How health care services are accessed, delivered, evaluated and financed is dependent on a confluence of factors, including the social, cultural, economic, educational and environmental variables existing within any community. The tri-county area represents the most diverse region in Indiana, and its health care profile reflects this profile. Health care coverage for Indiana residents is approximated to be 80%, less than the baseline of 86% and target of 100% coverage nationwide. The percentage of adult working poor without health care coverage

TABLE 2-1 The PROCESS of Health and Wellness Assessment

P urpose/Problem	Determine the **Purpose** of the assessment; define and describe the problem.
R efine	Formulate and **Refine** the primary questions and all associated questions of the assessment study.
O rganize	**Organize** the coalition to identify, retrieve, and categorize data.
C ompare	**Compare** the information against the *Healthy People 2010* benchmarks. These benchmarks provide a standard for measurement of quality health care.
E valuate	**Evaluate** the outcomes of existing health and wellness services by applying *Healthy People 2010* benchmarks to actual health and wellness outcomes.
S ummarize	**Summarize** findings and make recommendations.
S ubmit report	**Submit** the report.

is even larger. Although Northwest Indiana provides health care clinics that may provide free or pro-rated services, transportation to these clinics remains problematic, especially for the elderly and for pregnant and parenting adolescents.

Childhood immunization rates, although improving, still fall between 51% to 79% for the tri-county area. The early childhood vaccination rate for the state, at 72%, falls below the 76% rate for the nation. Half of older, non-institutionalized adults in Indiana are not vaccinated for influenza. Tri-county hospital discharge rates from asthma and bronchitis constitute 18% of total discharge rates in the state for this condition, which reflects the problem of chronic pulmonary conditions for this region. Asthma still affects 17% of all Indiana schoolchildren. Other chronic health conditions, which can be prevented or ameliorated through primary care, still account for a sizeable amount of unemployment or physical limitations in Indiana adults.

Approximately one-fourth of Indiana adults have already lost six or more teeth due to decay or gum disease, which reflects either lack of access to preventative dental care or lack of educational services related to good dental health. More than a third of Indiana adults had not visited a dentist or dental clinic within a year. Although the IUN School of Dental Education affiliates with Gary Community Health

Center to offer an oral health program to its clients, the population served remains small, and its services are limited. (Nardi, Sutherland, Strupeck, & Tippy, 2000, pp. 72–73).

EXAMPLE: *HEALTHY PEOPLE 2010* GOAL ONE: ACCESS TO CARE

The following example, used with permission from a health and wellness needs assessment for a Midwestern region, conducted by a research team of faculty, community leaders, and health care providers, summarizes the steps of their assessment using the Ontario Needs Impact Based Model:

Three types of needs are examined: normative, comparative, felt and expressed, to determine the health and wellness needs for Northwest Indiana. Normative needs are the benchmarks described by *Healthy People 2010*. Indicators of comparative needs include data regarding the determinants of health for the population of the three major counties served by Indiana University Northwest: Lake, Porter and La Porte. Expressed needs related to health are gathered from selected key informants, who are the users and providers of health care and community services in the Northwest Indiana area. Needs assessment questions were developed using the *Healthy People 2010* leading health indicators as the national standards for health and wellness. Information was collected using interviews, focus groups and a secondary analysis of official documents reporting the most current health and wellness statistical data for the counties of Lake, Porter and La Porte counties. This data was compared with leading health indicators, and levels of needs were categorized by service-related or evaluation/research related needs. These leading health indicators also inform any subsequent planning to address identified health and wellness service and evaluation/research needs. (Nardi, Sutherland, Strupeck, & Tippy, 2000, p. 13)

DEVELOPING A NEEDS ASSESSMENT TOOL

A needs assessment tool allows easy comparison of the data by category and results to any and all of the *Healthy People 2010* goals and objectives. The tool is a table labeled by the goal that is being addressed. There are 28 separate needs assessment tools, one for each goal, located on the companion web site, at http://www.delmarhealthcare.com, and they can be downloaded for use in categorizing and comparing assessment data. The table consists of six columns, and the number of rows corresponds with the number of objectives listed under each goal. For instance, the number of rows for *Goal One: Access to Care*, is 13, one row for each of its 13 objectives; the number of rows for *Goal Eight: Environmental Health*, is 30, one for each of its 30 objectives. See Table 2-2.

The first row of the table presents the goal. The first two columns contain the numbered objectives and target benchmarks for each. The other three columns are used to compare the related data to the benchmarks, to determine if a need exists, and to develop recommendations appropriate to the identified need. If a need exists, the column is marked with an *X;* if no need exists, the column is left unmarked. If there is not enough data to make a determination of need, a ? is used to signify that more data, or data specific to *Healthy People 2010* benchmarks, is needed to determine need. Table 2-2 presents the results of this assessment of access to care in the community, categorized by Leading Health Indicators as numbered objectives, as well as comparative data, identified needs, and recommendations. The data concerning this one goal indicates that all relevant objectives have not been met, either because a need is clearly indicated or because the indicated data is not readily available to the assessment team. This comparison between the objective-related data and the target benchmarks assists the assessment team in identifying health and wellness needs in this area, and in taking steps to form recommendations to address the need. This tool is an example for demonstration purposes only, and does not include all 13 objectives that *Healthy Person 2010* goal 1 comprises. The developmental objectives, which do not specify target benchmarks, are not included. Developmental objectives are those that were deemed important enough to drive assessment and implementation, but are not supported by data from a national surveillance system data.

When the assessment team uses goal-related *Healthy People 2010* objectives that are termed "developmental," benchmarks can be established based on the evidence contained in the literature, or from key informant testimony. For instance, the second objective under *Goal One: Access to Care* is developmental. It addresses the need to increase the proportion of insured people with coverage for clinical preventive services. Clinical preventive services include such programs as stop-smoking programs at work and well-child programs. After a review of the literature on clinical preventive services or well-child programs, the assessment team might include this objective and set a benchmark of 100 percent coverage of well-child programs for all work-related insurance programs for businesses with over 100 employees. Needs assessment tools for all 28 *Healthy People*

continuies on p. 43

TABLE 2-2 Needs Assessment Tool 1

Goal One: Improve access to comprehensive, high-quality health care services

HP 2010 OBJECTIVES	TARGET	DATA ASSESSED	NEED	RECOMMENDATIONS
1. Increase the proportion of persons with health insurance.	To 100%	During 1995, 12.1% (10,300) of NWI area adults did not have health care insurance; 5.6% of area people living in poverty did not have health care insurance (PRC Community health Assessment, 1996).	X	Develop a regional health and wellness center, affiliated with area hospitals, to meet primary health needs of the underserved
4. Increase the proportion of persons who have a age specific source of ongoing care.	To 96% for all ages			
5. Increase the proportion of persons with a usual primary care provider.	To 85%			
6. Reduce the proportion of families that experience difficulties or delays in obtaining health care or do not receive needed care for one or more family members.	To 7%			

continues

TABLE 2-2 Needs Assessment Tool 1 *continued*

Goal One: Improve access to comprehensive, high-quality health care services

HP 2010 OBJECTIVES	TARGET	DATA ASSESSED	NEED	RECOMMENDATIONS
8. In the health professions, allied and associated health profession fields, and the nursing field, increase the proportion of all degrees awarded to members of under-represented racial and ethnic groups.	To 1–13% (see specific target for each racial	About 3% of Indiana RN's are African American, 1% are Asian American, 0.2% are Native American, and 0.8% claim other racial groups (Indiana Health Care, 2000; Self-Study, 2000). About 60% of the 13,477 physicians holding an Indiana license had a practice located in Indiana. Of these, 82.2% were White, 2.9% were Black, and approx. 2% of Hispanic origin; 17% were women (Indiana Health Care Prof. Dev. Commission, 1998).	X	Funded secondary schools-college linkage program to encourage minority student enrollment and retention in health professions programs
9. Reduce hospitalization rates for three ambulatory-care-sensitive conditions; pediatric asthma, uncontrolled diabetes, and immunization-preventable pneumonia and influenza in older adults.	Admissions per 10,000 population Pediatric asthma to 17.3 < 18 yrs. Uncontrolled diabetes to 5.3 18–64 yrs.	In Gary, IN, in 1997, Diabetes Mellitus was the fifth leading cause of death for all; the fifth leading cause of death for males, the fourth leading cause of death for females, the fourth leading cause of death for whites and the fifth leading cause of death for blacks; the fourth leading cause of death for white males; the fifth leading cause of death for black males; the fourth leading cause of death for black females (Data and Stats, 1997).	X	Service-learning programs in health professions schools to offer health education/primary prevention, stop smoking and immunization programs at parent groups, churches and schools.

Immunization-preventable pneumonia or influenza > 65		In 1998, 50.1% of older adults, non-institutionalized, high-risk age 65 and older had never received a pneumococcal vaccination (Healthy People 2000 in Indiana, 2000). Some form of asthma affects 17% of all school age children in Indiana (Indiana State Department of Health, 2000).		
12. Establish a single toll-free telephone number for access to poison control centers on a 24-hour basis throughout the United States.	To 100%	The Northwest Indiana region is served by a statewide poison control center, open 24 hours per day that has been in existence since 1989. It is located in the Methodist Hospitals in Indianapolis. The toll-free number is 1-800-382-9097. There are no plans at this time to merge services with a national center (Indiana Poison Control Center, personal interview, September 5, 2000).		
13. Increase outcomes of [States] with trauma care systems that maximize outcomes of trauma patients and help prevent injuries from occurring.	Total coverage	No data available	?	Study on effectiveness of trauma care systems in the NW Indiana area

continues

TABLE 2-2 Needs Assessment Tool 1 *continued*

Goal One: Improve access to comprehensive, high-quality health care services

HP 2010 OBJECTIVES	TARGET	DATA ASSESSED	NEED	RECOMMENDATIONS
14. Increase the number of States . . . that have implemented guidelines for prehospital and hospital pediatric care.	All states	The FDA has estimated that there are 50,000 to 60,000 user facilities that require training on when and how they should report device-related events. Consequently, the FDA does not have the resources to train personnel or the resources to routinely monitor the user facilities' device-related reporting patterns. A proposed solution is a sentinel surveillance system (U.S. Food and Drug Administration, 1999)	X	Study of use of standardized guidelines for prehospital and hospital pediatric care.
16. Reduce the proportion of nursing home residents with a current diagnosis of pressure ulcers.	8 diagnoses per 1,000 residents	No data available	?	Re-examine identification of data sources and data collection methods

2010 goals with a complete list of their objectives are located on the companion web site, and can be downloaded for use in identifying, categorizing, comparing, and applying health and wellness assessment data.

 ## KEY POINTS

- ◆ Before beginning, informed consent must be obtained when collecting primary data through individual interviews or when conducting focus groups or surveys.

- ◆ The first step of a health and wellness needs assessment is to decide why you need to do one, explain the problem, describe your purpose, and identify the area or group to be assessed.

- ◆ The purpose of a needs assessment can be determined by posing a question about health and wellness that arises from personal experience or through a literature review.

- ◆ Creating community investment in the needs assessment is key to its success in obtaining agency and key informant cooperation when gathering relevant data and implementing any recommendations derived from the assessment.

- ◆ A coalition of individuals who are cooperating to conduct a needs assessment can accomplish a health and wellness needs assessment more effectively than one person working alone.

- ◆ The steps of coalition building are: (1) define goals and objectives; (2) identify the problem; (3) engage community leaders or interested parties who would want to be involved; (4) maintain the coalition.

- ◆ A conceptual framework can serve as a road map for choosing the areas of health and wellness related to the concerns that should be assessed, and for identifying the information required to do so.

- ◆ Primary and secondary sources are used to gather information. The goal of information gathering is to obtain useful data about the community and its health and wellness needs.

- ◆ Information about the community's expressed needs and felt needs can serve to inform and validate any data that team is also collecting through secondary means. These needs can be compared to *Healthy People 2010* normative needs to determine comparative needs.

- The first step in the analysis process is to examine the data for any omissions, mislabeling or errors before going any further.

- The second step in the analysis process is to categorize the data according to selected *Healthy People 2010* objectives.

- The third step in the analysis process is to compare the data by using a needs assessment tool to the related *Healthy People 2010* benchmarks to determine if a need exists or if the target has been met for that item.

- Finally, logical conclusions can be drawn from the results of this comparison and then used to develop recommendations.

 REFERENCES

Allender, J., & Spradley, B. (2001). *Community health nursing: Concepts and practice* (3rd ed.). Philadelphia: Lippincott.

American Medical Association. (2000). *Code of medical ethics: Current opinions with annotations* (1998–1999 ed.). Chicago: American Medical Association.

American Nurses Association. (1997). *Code for nurses with interpretive statements.* Kansas City, MO: American Nurses Association.

Andersen, E. & McFarlane, (2000). *Community as partner* (4th ed.). Philadelphia: Lippincott.

Aspen Reference Group. (1997). Community health education and promotion: A guide to program design and evaluation. Gaithersburg, MD: Aspen Publishing.

Aydelotte, M. (1983). The future health care delivery system in the United States. In N. Chaska (Ed.), *The nursing profession: A time to speak.* New York: McGraw-Hill.

Burkhardt, M., & Nathaniel, A. (1998). *Ethics & issues in contemporary nursing.* Clifton Park, NY: Delmar Learning.

Cherry, B., & Jacob, S. (1999). *Contemporary nursing: Issues, trends & management.* St. Louis: Mosby.

Chitty, K. (2001). *Professional nursing: Concepts & challenges* (3rd ed.). Philadelphia: W. B. Saunders.

Data and stats. (2000) [online]. Available: http://www.stats.indiana.edu/.

Frisch, N., & Frisch, L. (2002). *Psychiatric mental health nursing* (2nd ed.). Clifton Park, NY: Delmar Learning.

Healthy People 2000 in Indiana. (1998). *Report on progress Healthy People 2000.* Available: stats/brffs/1998/app_a_table.htm.

Indiana Health Care Professional Development Commission. (1998). *Annual report. Indiana State Department of Health* [online]. Available: http://www.state.in.us/isdh/publications/1998report.

Indiana State Department of Health. (2000). 1999 *Indiana report of diseases of public health interest* [online]. Available: http://www.state.in.us/isdh/dataandstats/disease/1999/index.htm

Indiana State Department of Health (2000). *Indiana health behavior risk factors report 1998 state data, 1997.* Indianapolis: Indiana State Department of Health.

L, NT. (2000). ADE rate uncertain, reporting systems inadequate, GAO tells legislators. *American Journal of Health-System Pharmacy, 57*(6), 515–516, 519.

Lundy, K., & Janes, S. (2001). *Community health nursing: Caring for the public's health.* Sudbury, MA: Jones and Bartlett.

McBride, A. (2000). Interesting facts [electronic mail] [online]. Available: amcmcbride@iupui.edu.

Nardi, D., Sutherland, T., Tippy, F., & Strupeck, D. (Eds.). (2000). *Needs assessment of the health and wellbeing of Northwest Indiana.* Indiana University Northwest, Shared Vision Research and Service Task Forces. Unpublished manuscript.

Patton, M. (1990). *Qualitative evaluation and research methods.* Newbury Park: Sage Publications.

Physicians for a National Health Program: PNHP. (2000, September). *PHNP newsletter.* Chicago: PHNP.

PRC Community Health Assessment. (1996). *Merrillville, Gary, IN.* Omaha, NE: Professional Research Consultants, Inc.

Rodeghier, M. (1996). *Surveys with confidence: A practical guide to survey research using SPSS.* Chicago: SPSS.

Schutt, R. (1999). Investigating the social world: The process and practice of research (2nd ed.). Thousand Oaks, CA: Pine Forge Press.

Schutt, R. (2001). Investigating the social world: The process and practice of research. (3rd ed.). Boston: Pine Forge Press.

Strauss, A. (2000). *Qualitative analysis for social scientists.* Cambridge: Cambridge University Press.

Sultz, H., & Young, K. (1999). *Health care USA: Understanding its organization and delivery.* Gathersburg, MD: Aspen Publications.

U.S. Department of Health and Human Services. (2000, January). *Healthy People 2010.* (Conference Edition, in Two Volumes). Washington, DC.

U.S. Food and Drug Administration—Center for Devices and Radiological Health. (2000). *Final report of a study to evaluate the feasibility and effectiveness of a sentinel reporting system for adverse event reporting of medical device use in user facilities, June 16, 1999* [online]. Available: http://www.fda.gov/cdrh/postsurv/medsunappendixa.html.

U.S. Preventative Services Task Force. (1996). *Guide to clinical preventative services* (2nd ed.). Baltimore: Williams & Wilkins.

Wandersman, A., Goodman, R., & Butterfoss, F. (1997). Understanding coalitions and how they operate: An "open system" organizational framework. In M. Minkler (Ed.), *Community organizing & community building for health.* New Brunswick, NJ: Rutgers University Press.

Chapter

3

ASSESSING PHYSICAL HEALTH AND WELLNESS

Charlene Gyurko

 LEARNING OBJECTIVES

At the conclusion of this chapter, the reader will be able to:

◆ Explain how the indicators of *Healthy People 2010* can be used to assess aspects of the community's physical health and wellness.

◆ Apply the Ontario Needs Impact Based Model to the assessment of health and wellness needs.

◆ Identify secondary data resources used to assess targeted community physical health and wellness needs.

◆ Recognize the interrelationships of disease processes.

◆ Compare and contrast primary, secondary, and tertiary health care utilization.

◆ Explain the relationship between Suchman's Stages of Illness Experience Model and *Healthy People 2010* goals.

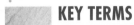 **KEY TERMS**

Acute disease	Infectious diseases
Cardiovascular	Multisystem disease process
Chronic disease	Primary health care
Human immunodeficiency virus (HIV)	Secondary health care
	Tertiary health care
Illness behavior	

I n this chapter, the steps of health and well-being needs assessment are applied to actual physical health and wellness issues using secondary data analysis methodology, as described in Chapter 1. Representational data related to nine *Healthy People 2010* goals and their related objectives are selectively examined and compared to the objectives for understanding and improving the nation's health. The gathering and grouping of data concerning each of the nine goals is described. The sample needs assessment tool at the end of this chapter uses the Ontario Needs Impact Based Model to assess a region's needs related to *Healthy People 2010* goal 12: "Improve cardiovascular health and quality of life through the prevention, detection, and treatment of risk factors; early identification and treatment of heart attacks and strokes; and prevention of recent cardiovascular events." The term **cardiovascular** refers to the heart and its structures and related vasculature.

BEFORE BEGINNING: WHY THE NEED?

It goes without saying that health status is directly correlated with health behavior. Health behavior relates to the availability of health services. The availability of health services, in turn, is dependent upon employers, third-party payers such as traditional private insurers, managed care organizations, and government and state programs such as Medicare, Medicaid, and CHIPs. CHIP is the acronym for Children's Health Insurance Program. CHIP was created by Congress in 1997 as part of the federal balanced budget (CHIP—Children's Health Insurance Program, 1997). Free standing health care clinics are also becoming more prevalent throughout the United States.

The health status of a person directly parallels quality of life. *Healthy People* endeavors to improve the health of the nation, in particular, the federal, state, and local public health community (Healthy People 2000: Priority Areas and Area Resources, 2000). *Healthy People 2010* is consistent with that goal, since it continues to emphasize individual uses of private and public resources to live a healthier lifestyle. However, health insurance increases the individual's ability to access health and wellness resources (see Box 3-1). The numbers of uninsured when Medicare and Medicaid were passed in the 1960s is comparable to the current situation, in which over 43 million Americans presently lack health insurance. Between 1990 and 1999, the number of uninsured increased by 8 million. Of those without coverage, three-quarters are children and working adults. There is no current linkage between coverage and employment. Health insurance in the United States is not a right of citizenship (Himmelstein, Woolhandler, & Hellander, 2001).

By 1996, several million women and children had lost Medicaid coverage when welfare rolls were reduced (Harrington & Estes, 2001). In 1999, 40 percent of the 42.6 million uninsured Americans were without coverage for a period of at least three years

> **Box 3-1** ■ **Individual Responsibility for Health and Wellness**
>
> *In the United States, for example, the structural power of corporate and medical professional interests results in individual responsibility for health being defined in terms of consumer and life style behavior. The "responsible" person thus, is one who buys sufficient health insurance, consumes the right diet and avoids consuming the wrong products, purchases health professional care wisely, takes prescribed medications and complies with other "doctors-orders," spends stress-reducing vacations, and invests in a good health spa*
>
> —Donahue & McGuire, 1995, p. 48, in Matcha, 2000, p. 107

(Physicians for a National Health Program, 2001). The above data and criteria provide an important context, since all physical health and wellness needs are addressed in our society by services that are funded through private, state, federal, for-profit, not-for-profit, or nonprofit means.

STEPS OF THE PHYSICAL HEALTH AND WELL-BEING ASSESSMENT

Nine goals of *Healthy People 2010* address the assessment and functioning of overall physical health and wellness. Many of these goals demonstrate the interrelationship of chronic disease processes. A **chronic**

disease is slow in onset and lifelong in consequences; it cannot be cured but can be controlled. A person may have many chronic diseases and yet feel relatively healthy. The treatment may be extensive, however, and can be catastrophic in cost due to the diseases' exacerbations or recurrence. When a client with a chronic disease becomes ill, she or he is usually sicker than the client who does not have a chronic disease. Therefore, because the client with a chronic disease is already sick or debilitated because of the preexisting condition, it takes longer for the person to get better when a recurrence of that disease process occurs. Conversely, an **acute disease** is a disease having a sudden onset. Table 3-1 presents these nine goals, the general topics or issues addressed, and their relationship to related *Healthy People 2010* goals and objectives.

Information concerning the national status of efforts to achieve each goal is presented in order to explain the role the goal plays in the overall status of the physical health of the nation.

Step One: Definition and Description of the Needs Assessment Problem

The World Health Organization defines health and well-being as "a state of complete physical, social and mental well-being, and not merely the absence of disease or infirmity. . . . Health is a resource for everyday life, not the object of living. It is a positive concept emphasizing social and personal resources as well as physical capabilities" (World Health Organization, 2001, p. 1).

Health care professionals use this definition in the context of a holistic approach to assessing, delivering, and evaluating health care. Included are the interrelationships of physical, mental, spiritual, and psychosocial well-being of the client. In essence, a positive mental state seems to enhance the physical status or well-being of the person. Psychosocial well-being also seems to be related to a positive mental status. A positive spiritual well-being seems to enhance the physical and mental status of the client.

For the client with a chronic multisystem disease process, such as the cardiac client, well-being seems to be associated with stability of the disease process. A **multisystem disease process** is defined as a myriad of diseases in which more than one organ or bodily system is affected. This is due to the interrelationships of the malfunctioning organ with other organs. Considering that the heart carries blood and the blood carries oxygen, a person with heart disease can be said to be in a state of equilibrium or homeostasis from a physical, social, and mental well-being status from the mere fact that the client, from his or her own perception, feels good. It stands to reason that when one feels good, social and personal affect and physical capabilities seem to be enhanced.

TABLE 3-1 Most Common Categories of Theoretical Models

GOAL #	GENERAL TOPIC	HEALTHY PEOPLE 2010 GOAL	RELATED HEALTHY PEOPLE OBJECTIVES
2	Arthritis, other rheumatic and chronic conditions	Improve illness and disability related to arthritis and other rheumatic conditions, osteoporisis, and chronic back conditions.	*Access to Quality Health Services* 1–3. Counseling about health behaviors Cancer 3–10. Provider counseling about preventive measures Disability and Secondary Conditions 6–4. Social participation among adults with disabilities 6–5. Sufficient emotional support among adults with disabilities 6–8. Employment parity *Education and Community-Based Programs* 7–5. Worksite health promotion programs 7–6. Participation in employer-sponsored health promotion activities 7–10. Community health promotion programs 7–12. Older adult participation in community health promotion activities *Injury and Violence Prevention* 15–28. Hip fractures *Nutrition and Overweight* 19–1. Healthy weight in adults 19–2. Obesity in adults 19–11. Calcium intake

continues

TABLE 3-1 Most Common Categories of Theoretical Models *continued*

GOAL #	GENERAL TOPIC	HEALTHY PEOPLE 2010 GOAL	RELATED HEALTHY PEOPLE OBJECTIVES
			19–16. Worksite promotion of nutrition education and weight management
			19–17. Nutrition counseling for medical conditions
			Occupational Safety and Health
			20–2. Work-related injuries
			20–3. Overexertion or repetitive motion
			Physical Activity and Fitness
			22–1. No leisure-time physical extivity
			22–2. Moderate physical activity
			22–3. Vigorous physical activity
			22–4. Muscular strength and endurance
			22–5. Flexibility
			22–8. Physical education requirements in schools
			22–10. Physical activity in physical education class
			Tobacco Use
			27–1. Adult tobacco use
			27–5. Smoking cessation by adults
			27–7. Smoking cessation by adolescents
			27–17. Adolescent disapproval of smoking
3	Cancer	Reduce the number of new cancer cases as well as the illness, disability and death caused by cancer.	*Nutrition and Overweight*
			19–5. Fruit intake
			19–6. Vegetable intake
			19–8. Saturated fat intake
			19–9. Total fat intake

continues

| 4 | Chronic kidney disease | Reduce new cases of chronic kidney disease and its complication, disability, death and economic costs. | *Oral Health*
21-6. Early detection of oral and pharyngeal cancer
21-17. Annual examinations for oral and pharyngeal cancer
Tobacco Use
27-1. Adult tobacco use
27-2. Youth tobacco use
27-5. Smoking cessation by adults
27-7. Smoking cessation by adolescents
27-8. Insurance coverage of cessation treatment
Access to Quality Health Services
1-2. Health insurance coverage for clinical preventive services
1-3. Counseling about health behaviors
1-7. Core competencies in health provider training
Diabetes
5-2. Prevent diabetes
5-3. Reduce diabetes
5-4. Diagnosis of diabetes
5-7. Cardiovascular deaths in persons with diabetes
5-11. Annual urinary microalbumin measurement
5-12. Annual glycosylated hemoglobin measurement
Disability and Secondary Conditions
6-1. Standard definition of people with disabilities in data sets |

TABLE 3-1 Most Common Categories of Theoretical Models *continued*

GOAL #	GENERAL TOPIC	HEALTHY PEOPLE 2010 GOAL	RELATED HEALTHY PEOPLE OBJECTIVES
			6–2. Feelings and depression among children with disabilities
			6–3. Feelings and depression interfering with activities among adults with disabilities
			6–5. Sufficient emotional support among adults with disabilities
			6–6. Satisfaction with life among adults with disabilities
			6–8. Employment parity
			Educational and Community-Based Programs
			7–7. Patient and family education
			7–8. Satisfaction with patient education
			7–9. Health care organization sponsorship of community health promotion activities
			7–10. Community health promotion programs
			7–11. Culturally appropriate community health promotion programs
			Environmental Health
			8–11. Elevated blood lead levels in children
			8–14. Toxic pollutants
			8–20. School policies to protect against environmental hazards
			8–22. Lead-based paint testing
			8–25. Exposure to heavy metals and other toxic chemicals

8–26. Information systems used for environmental health
8–27. Monitoring environmentally related diseases
8–29. Global burden of disease

Food Safety
10–1. Foodborne infections
10–2. Outbreaks of foodborne infections
10–5. Consumer food safety practices
10–6. Safe food preparation practices in retail establishments

Health Communication
11–2. Health literacy
11–4. Quality of Internet health information sources
11–6. Satisfaction with providers' communication skills

Heart Disease and Stroke
12–1. Coronary heart disease (CHD) deaths
12–2. Knowledge of symptoms of heart attack and importance of dialing 911
12–6. Heart failure hospitalizations
12–8. Knowledge of early warning symptoms of stroke
12–9. High blood pressure
12–10. High blood pressure control
12–11. Action to help control blood pressure
12–12. Blood pressure monitoring
12–16. LDL-cholesterol level in CHD patients

HIV
13–1. New AIDS cases
13–3. AIDS cases among persons who inject drugs

continues

TABLE 3-1   Most Common Categories of Theoretical Models   *continued*

GOAL #	GENERAL TOPIC	HEALTHY PEOPLE 2010 GOAL	RELATED HEALTHY PEOPLE OBJECTIVES
			13–5. New HIV cases
			13–8. HIV counseling and education for persons in substance abuse treatment
			13–12. Screening for STDs and immunization for hepatitis B
			13–17. Perinatally acquired HIV infection
			Immunization and Infectious Diseases
			14–1. Vaccine-preventable diseases
			14–2. Hepatitis B in infants and young children
			14–3. Hepatitis B in adults and high-risk groups
			14–9. Hepatitis C
			14–10. Identification of persons with chronic hepatitis C
			14–16. Invasive early-onset group B streptococcal disease
			14–28. Hepatitis B vaccination among high-risk groups
			Maternal, Infant, and Child Health
			16–10. Low birth weight and very low birth weight
			Medical Product Safety
			17–1. Monitoring of adverse medical events
			17–2. Linked, automated information systems
			17–3. Provider review of medications taken by patients
			17–6. Blood donations
			Nutrition and Overweight
			19–1. Healthy weight in adults
			19–2. Obesity in adults

19–8. Saturated fat intake

19–17. Nutrition counseling for medical conditions

Occupational Safety and Health

20–7. Elevated blood lead levels from work exposure

Physical Activity and Fitness

22–2. Moderate physical activity

22–3. Vigorous physical activity

22–13. Worksite physical activity and fitness

Public Health Infrastructure

23–2. Public access to information and surveillance data

23–3. Use of geocoding in health data systems

23–4. Data for all population groups

23–5. Data for Leading Health Indicators, Health Status Indicators, and Priority Data Needs at State, Tribal, and local levels

23–6. National tracking of Healthy People 2010 objectives

23–7. Timely release of data on objectives

23–17. Prevention research

Sexually Transmitted Diseases

25–3. Primary and secondary syphilis

25–8. Heterosexually transmitted HIV infection in women

25–10. Neonatal STDs

25–13. Hepatitis B vaccine services in STD clinics

Tobacco Use

27–1. Adult tobacco use

27–2. Adolescent tobacco use

27–5. Smoking cessation by adults

continues

TABLE 3-1 Most Common Categories of Theoretical Models *continued*

GOAL #	GENERAL TOPIC	HEALTHY PEOPLE 2010 GOAL	RELATED HEALTHY PEOPLE OBJECTIVES
5	Diabetes	Through prevention programs, reduce the disease and economic burden of diabetes and improve the quality of life for all persons who have or at risk for diabetes.	27-7. Smoking cessation by adolescents 27-10. Exposure to environmental tobacco smoke *Access to Quality Health Services* 1-1. Persons with health insurance 1-2. Health insurance coverage for clinical preventive services 1-3. Counseling about health behaviors *Chronic Kidney Disease* 4-1. End-stage renal disease 4-2. Cardiovascular disease deaths in persons with chronic kidney failure 4-7. Kidney failure due to diabetes 4-8. Medical therapy for persons with diabetes and proteinuria *Family Planning* 9-3. Contraceptive use 9-11. Pregnancy prevention education *Heart Disease and Stroke* 12-1. Coronary heart disease (CHD) deaths 12-2. Knowledge of symptoms of heart attack and importance of dialing 911 12-7. Stroke deaths 12-8. Knowledge of early warning symptoms of stroke 12-9. High blood pressure

12–10. High blood pressure control
12–11. Action to help control blood pressure
12–12. Blood pressure monitoring
12–13. Mean total cholesterol levels
12–14. High blood cholesterol levels
12–15. Blood cholesterol screening
12–16. LDL-cholesterol level in CHD patients

Immunization and Infectious Diseases
14–5. Invasive pneumococcal infections
14–29. Flu and pneumococcal vaccination of high-risk adults

Maternal, Infant, and Child Health
16–6. Prenatal care
16–10. Low birth weight and very low birth weight
16–19. Breastfeeding

Nutrition and Overweight
19–1. Healthy weight in adults
19–2. Obesity in adults
19–3. Overweight or obesity in children and adolescents
19–16. Worksite promotion of nutrition education and weight management
19–17. Nutrition counseling for medical conditions

Physical Activity and Fitness
22–1. No leisure-time physical activity
22–2. Moderate physical activity
22–3. Vigorous physical activity

continues

TABLE 3-1 Most Common Categories of Theoretical Models *continued*

GOAL #	GENERAL TOPIC	HEALTHY PEOPLE 2010 GOAL	RELATED HEALTHY PEOPLE OBJECTIVES
			22–6. Moderate physical activity in adolescents
			22–7. Vigorous physical activity in adolescents
			Vision and Hearing
			28–1. Dilated eye exam
			28–5. Impairment due to diabetic retinopathy
			28–10. Vision rehabilitation services and devices
12	Cardiovascular health	Improve cardiovascular health and quality of life through prevention, detection and treatment of risk factors; early identification and treatment of heart attacks and strokes; and prevention of recurrent cardiovascular events.	*Access to Quality Health Services*
			1–2. Health insurance coverage for clinical preventive services
			1–3. Counseling about health behaviors
			1–7. Core competencies in health provider training
			Diabetes
			5–2. Prevent diabetes
			5–3. Reduce diabetes
			5–4. Diagnosis of diabetes
			5–7. Cardiovascular deaths in persons with diabetes
			5–11. Annual urinary microalbumin measurement
			5–12. Annual glycosylated hemoglobin measurement
			Disability and Secondary Conditions
			6–1. Standard definition of people with disabilities in data sets
			6–2. Feelings and depression among children with disabilities
			6–3. Feelings and depression interfering with activities among adults with disabilities

6–5. Sufficient emotional support among adults with disabilities

6–6. Satisfaction with life among adults with disabilities

6–8. Employment parity

Educational and Community-Based Programs

7–7. Patient and family education

7–8. Satisfaction with patient education

7–9. Health care organization sponsorship of community health promotion activities

7–10. Community health promotion programs

7–11. Culturally appropriate community health promotion programs

Environmental Health

8–11. Elevated blood lead levels in children

8–15. Toxic pollutants

8–20. School policies to protect against environmental hazards

8–22. Lead-based paint testing

8–25 Exposure to heavy metals and other toxic chemicals

8–26. Information systems used for environmental health

8–27. Monitoring environmentally related diseases

8–29. Global burden of disease

Food Safety

10–1. Foodborne infections

10–2. Outbreaks of foodborne infections

10–5. Consumer food safety practices

10–6 Safe food preparation practices in retail establishments

continues

TABLE 3-1 Most Common Categories of Theoretical Models *continued*

GOAL #	GENERAL TOPIC	HEALTHY PEOPLE 2010 GOAL	RELATED HEALTHY PEOPLE OBJECTIVES
			Health Communication
			11–2. Health literacy
			11–4. Quality of Internet health information sources
			11–6. Satisfaction with providers' communication skills
			Heart Disease and Stroke
			12–1. Coronary heart disease (CHD) deaths
			12–2. Knowledge of symptoms of heart attack and importance of dialing 911
			12–6. Heart failure hospitalizations
			12–8. Knowledge of early warning symptoms of stroke
			12–9. High blood pressure
			12–10. High blood pressure control
			12–11. Action to help control blood pressure
			12–12. Blood pressure monitoring
			12–16. LDL-cholesterol level in CHD patients
			HIV
			13–1. New AIDS cases
			13–3. AIDS cases among persons who inject drugs
			13–5. New HIV cases
			13–8. HIV counseling and education for persons in substance abuse treatment
			13–12. Screening for STDs and immunization for hepatitis B
			13–17. Perinatally acquired HIV infection

continues

TABLE 3-1 Most Common Categories of Theoretical Models *continued*

GOAL #	GENERAL TOPIC	HEALTHY PEOPLE 2010 GOAL	RELATED HEALTHY PEOPLE OBJECTIVES
			Public Health Infrastructure
			23–2. Public access to information and surveillance data
			23–3. Use of geocoding in health data systems
			23–4. Data for all population groups
			23–5. Data for Leading Health Indicators, Health Status Indicators, and Priority Data Needs at State, Tribal, and local levels
			23–6. National tracking of Healthy People 2010 objectives
			23–7. Timely release of data on objectives
			23–17. Prevention research
			Sexually Transmitted Diseases
			25–3. Primary and secondary syphilis
			25–8. Heterosexually transmitted HIV infection in women
			25–11. Neonatal STDs
			25–13. Hepatitis B vaccine services in STD clinics
			Tobacco Use
			27–1. Adult tobacco use
			27–2. Adolescent tobacco use
			27–5. Smoking cessation by adults
			27–7. Smoking cessation by adolescents
			27–10. Exposure to environmental tobacco smoke

| 19 | Diet and exercise | Promote health and reduce chronic disease associated with diet and weight. | *Access to Quality Health Services*
1–3. Counseling about health behaviors
Arthritis, Osteoporosis, and Chronic Back Conditions
2–9. Cases of osteoporosis
Cancer
3–1. Cancer deaths
3–3. Breast cancer deaths
3–5. Colorectal cancer deaths
3–10. Provider counseling about preventive measures
Chronic Kidney Disease
4–3. Counseling for chronic kidney failure care
Diabetes
5–1. Diabetes education
5–2. Prevent diabetes
5–6. Diabetes-related deaths
Educational and Community-Based Programs
7–2. School health education
7–5. Worksite health promotion programs
7–6. Participation in employer-sponsored health promotion activities
7–10. Community health promotion programs
7–11. Culturally appropriate community health promotion programs
Food Safety
10–4. Food allergy deaths
10–5. Consumer food safety practices |

continues

TABLE 3-1 Most Common Categories of Theoretical Models *continued*

GOAL #	GENERAL TOPIC	HEALTHY PEOPLE 2010 GOAL	RELATED HEALTHY PEOPLE OBJECTIVES
			Health Communication
			11–4. Quality of Internet health information sources
			Diabetes Heart Disease and Stroke
			12–1. Coronary heart disease (CHD) deaths
			12–7. Stroke deaths
			12–9. High blood pressure
			12–11. Action to help control blood pressure
			12–13. Mean total cholesterol levels
			12–14. High blood cholesterol levels
			Maternal, Infant, and Child Health
			16–10. Low birth weight and very low birth weight
			16–12- Weight gain during pregnancy
			16–15- Spina bifida and other neural tube defects
			16–16. Optimum folic acid
			16–17. Prenatal substance exposure
			16–18. Fetal alcohol syndrome
			16–19. Breastfeeding
			Mental Health and Mental Disorders
			18–5. Eating disorder relapses
			Physical Activity and Fitness
			22–1. No leisure-time physical activity
			22–2. Moderate physical activity
			22–3. Vigorous physical activity
			22–6. Moderate physical activity in adolescents

continues

| 21 | Dental and craniofacial health | Prevent and control oral and craniofacial diseases, conditions, and injuries and improve access to related services. | 22–7. Vigorous physical activity in adolescents
22–9. Daily physical education in schools
22–13. Worksite physical activity and fitness
Substance Abuse
26–12. Average annual alcohol consumption

Access to Quality Health Services
1–1. Persons with health insurance
1–2. Health insurance coverage for clinical preventive services
1–3. Counseling about health behaviors
1–4. Source of ongoing care
1–7. Core competencies in health provider training
1–8. Racial and ethnic representation in health professions
1–15. Long-term care services
Arthritis, Osteoporosis, and Chronic Back Conditions
2–2. Activity limitations due to arthritis
2–3. Personal care limitations
2–7. Seeing a health care provider
2–8. Arthritis education
Cancer
3–1. Cancer deaths
3–6. Oropharyngeal cancer deaths
3–9. Sun exposure
3–10. Provider counseling about preventive measures
3–14. Statewide cancer registries
3–15. Cancer survival rates |

TABLE 3-1 Most Common Categories of Theoretical Models *continued*

GOAL #	GENERAL TOPIC	HEALTHY PEOPLE 2010 GOAL	RELATED HEALTHY PEOPLE OBJECTIVES
			Diabetes
			5-1. Diabetes education
			5-2. Prevent diabetes
			5-3. Reduce diabetes
			5-4. Diagnosis of diabetes
			Disability and Secondary Conditions
			6-13. Surveillance and health promotion programs
			Educational and Community-Based Programs
			7-1. High school completion
			7-2. School health education
			7-3. Health-risk behavior information for college and university students
			7-4. School nurse-to-student ratio
			7-5. Worksite health promotion programs
			7-6. Participation in employer-sponsored health promotion activities
			7-7. Patient and family education
			7-10. Community health promotion programs
			7-11. Culturally appropriate community health promotion programs
			7-12. Older adult participation in community health promotion activities
			Environmental Health
			8-5. Safe drinking water

continues

Health Communication

11-1. Households with Internet access
11-2. Health literacy
11-3. Research and evaluation of communication programs
11-4. Quality of Internet health information sources
11-6. Satisfaction with providers' communication skills

Heart Disease and Stroke

12-1. Coronary heart disease (CHD) deaths

Immunization and Infectious Diseases

14-3. Hepatitis B in adults and high-risk groups
14-9. Hepatitis C
14-10. Identification of persons with chronic hepatitis C
14-28. Hepatitis B vaccination among high-risk groups

Injury and Violence Prevention

15-1. Nonfatal head injuries
15-17. Nonfatal motor vehicle injuries
15-19. Safety belts
15-20. Child restraints
15-21. Motorcycle helmet use
15-23. Bicycle helmet use
15-24. Bicycle helmet laws
15-31. Injury protection in school sports

Maternal, Infant, and Child Health

16-6. Prenatal care
16-8. Very low birth weight infants born at Level III hospitals

TABLE 3-1 Most Common Categories of Theoretical Models *continued*

GOAL #	GENERAL TOPIC	HEALTHY PEOPLE 2010 GOAL	RELATED HEALTHY PEOPLE OBJECTIVES
			16-10. Low birth weight and very low birth weight
			16-11. Preterm birth
			16-16. Optimum folic acid
			16-19. Breastfeeding
			16-23. Service systems for children with special health care needs
			Medical Product Safety
			17-3. Provider review of medications taken by patients
			17-4. Receipt of useful information from pharmacies
			17-5. Receipt of oral counseling from prescribers and dispensers
			Mental Health and Mental Disorders
			18-5. Eating disorder relapses
			Nutrition and Overweight
			19-1. Healthy weight in adults
			19-2. Obesity in adults
			19-3. Overweight and obesity in children and adolescents
			19-5. Fruit intake
			19-6. Vegetable intake
			19-11. Calcium intake
			19-15. Meals and snacks at school
			19-16. Worksite promotion of nutrition education and weight management

continues

TABLE 3-1 Most Common Categories of Theoretical Models *continued*

GOAL #	GENERAL TOPIC	HEALTHY PEOPLE 2010 GOAL	RELATED HEALTHY PEOPLE OBJECTIVES
			Substance Abuse 26–12. Average annual alcohol consumption *Tobacco Use* 27–1. Adult tobacco use 27–2 Adolescent tobacco use 27–3. Initiation of tobacco use 27–4. Age at first use of tobacco 27–5. Smoking cessation by adults 27–7. Smoking cessation by adolescents 27–8. Insurance coverage of cessation treatment 27–11. Smoke-free and tobacco-free schools 27–12. Worksite smoking policies 27–14. Enforcement of illegal tobacco sales to minors laws 27–15. Retail license suspension for sales to minors 27–18. Tobacco control programs 27–19. Preemptive tobacco control laws 27–20. Tobacco product regulation 27–21. Tobacco tax
24	Respiratory health	Promote respiratory health through better prevention, detection, treatment, and education.	*Access to Quality Health Services* 1–10. Delay or difficulty in getting emergency care *Educational and Community-Based Programs* 7–8. Satisfaction with patient education 7–10. Culturally appropriate community health promotion

Environmental Health

8–1. Harmful air pollutants

8–2. Alternative modes of transportation

8–3. Cleaner alternative fuels

8–4. Airborne toxins

8–14. Toxic pollutants

8–16. Indoor allergens

8–17. Office building air quality

8–20. School policies to protect against environmental hazards

8–23. Substandard housing

8–26. Information systems used for environmental health

8–27. Monitoring environmentally related diseases

8–28. Local agencies using surveillance data for vector control

Health Communication

11–6. Satisfaction with providers' communication skills

Injury and Violence Prevention

15–15. Deaths from motor vehicle crashes

15–17. Nonfatal motor vehicle injuries

Occupational Safety and Health

20–1. Work-related injury deaths

20–2. Work-related injuries

20–4. Pneumoconiosis deaths

Physical Activity and Fitness

22–6. Moderate physical activity in young persons

22–7. Vigorous physical activity in young people

continues

TABLE 3-1 Most Common Categories of Theoretical Models *continued*

GOAL #	GENERAL TOPIC	HEALTHY PEOPLE 2010 GOAL	RELATED HEALTHY PEOPLE OBJECTIVES
			Public Health Infrastructure
			23–2. Public access to information and surveillance data
			23–6. Data for all population groups
			23–6. National tracking of Healthy People 2010 objectives
			23–7. Timely release of data on objectives
			23–10. Continuing education and training by public health agencies
			23–16. Data on public health expenditures
			23–17. Prevention research
			Tobacco Use
			27–1. Adult tobacco use
			27–2. Adolescent tobacco use
			27–3. Initiation of tobacco use
			27–4. Age at first use of tobacco
			27–5. Smoking cessation by adults
			27–6. Smoking cessation during pregnancy
			27–7. Smoking cessation by adolescents
			27–8. Insurance coverage of cessation treatment
			27–9. Exposure to tobacco smoke at home among children
			27–10. Exposure to environmental tobacco smoke
			27–11. Smoke-free and tobacco-free schools
			27–12. Worksite smoking policies
			27–13. Smoke-free indoor air laws

| 28 | Vision and hearing | Improve the visual and hearing health of the Nation through prevention, early detection, treatment and rehabilitation. | 27–14. Enforcement of illegal tobacco sales to minors laws
27–15. Retail license suspension for sales to minors
27–16. Tobacco advertising and promotion targeting adolescents and young adults
27–17. Adolescent disapproval of smoking
27–18. Tobacco control programs
27–19. Preemptive tobacco control laws
27–20. Tobacco product regulation
27–21. Tobacco tax

Diabetes
5–13. Annual dilated eye examinations
Disability and Secondary Conditions
6–11. Assistive devices and technology
Occupational Safety and Health
20–11. Work-related, noise-induced hearing loss |

Source: Reprinted with permission from the U.S. Department of Health and Human Services. (2000, January). *Healthy People 2010* (Conference Edition, in Two Volumes). Washington, DC.

Examining the demographics of the environmental trends of the aging population, including poverty and social status, the 1960–1980 period revealed that the aging of the population was not an issue in determining well-being. However, infectious diseases posed the major health-related problems within this time frame. The 1980–2000 period exhibited an emergent issue in relation to the aging population as chronic diseases encompassed the bulk of the health care issues. *Healthy People 2000* focused on issues of heart disease and stroke, cancer, diabetes, and human immunodeficiency virus (HIV) infection. **Infectious diseases** are diseases that can be passed from one person to another by various means such as sputum, blood, body secretions, airborne mucous particles, and so on. Examples of infectious diseases listed include pneumonia, hepatitis, HIV, and tuberculosis. **Human immunodeficiency virus (HIV)** is a virus that is the causative agent of auto immune deficiency syndrome (AIDS). Not everyone who has HIV has AIDS, but everyone who has AIDS has HIV (Healthy People 2000: Priority Areas and Area Resources, 2001). The following description of the services provided by one church-based free health center illustrates how one organization began to address its identified health and wellness needs, which was to provide quality health care to the medically underserved in their community.

To address the health needs of the underinsured in one region of a Midwestern state, a church-affiliated health care center was formed in 1994. The purpose of this center was to offer health care in a free standing church-based clinic. During its inception, basic health services were provided to the community by means of local health fairs. Services were provided free of charge by students enrolled in affiliating health divisions and programs from a local college and state university. Free services in terms of blood draws for diabetic screening and HIV testing were also provided from the medical center, which was located in the city. The city's Board of Health provided free tuberculosis testing and readings in addition to well-baby and preschool immunizations. Blood pressure screenings specifically targeted young Black males. Massages, scoliosis screenings, nutritional assessments, dental screenings, and stress assessments were some of the other services the clinic offered through volunteerism and health fairs.

Step Two: Determining What Information Is Required

Health is just not a commodity of everyday living, it is a necessity. The population is aging. The proportion of persons age 65 and older grew from 10 percent to 13 percent between the years of 1970 and 1997 (Gallo, Fulmer, Paveze, et al., 2000). By 2050, those over age 65 are expected to make up 30 percent of the population, while the number of those over age 85 is expected to double. Those under age 35 are expected to comprise 10 percent of the total population (Sultz & Young, 2001). Those seeking medical assistance are often experiencing acute exacerbations of a chronic disease process. Therefore, they are usually more debilitated and incapacitated before seeking medical assistance, requiring more involved, more comprehensive, and more sustainable care.

To further address this issue, the cardiac client, or the person with a heart condition, will be discussed. When looking at a cardiac client, it must be noted that more than the heart is at stake. If the heart is damaged or weakened by a heart attack, a virus, or hypertension, the ultimate consequences are that the heart will not be able to pump adequate amounts of blood to the vital organs. Blood contains oxygen, and oxygen is a vital nutrient to all the cells of the body. Lack of oxygen will weaken the lungs and all of the other organs. One of the main organs affected are the kidneys. If the kidneys are damaged and shut down, the client experiences fluid overload, further increasing the amount of work that the heart must do. A common effect of this process is hypertension, or high blood pressure.

Decreased oxygen supply can also cause problems with cerebrovascular blood flow, with possible consequences of stroke (now more commonly defined as brain attack). To further compound the problem, if the heart can no longer pump adequately, the client can experience cardiogenic shock. With cardiogenic shock, all of the major body organs are affected in an acute manner, due to a chronic or ongoing problem that has suddenly worsened. In essence, even if the client feels good while taking prescribed medications or treatment for a chronic problem, the client will always experience some level of the persistent state of the disease process and some degree of damage to vital organs will always be present.

A cardiac arrhythmia is an abnormal and sometimes irregular heart beat. A significant complication of heart failure is an abnormal heartbeat called atrial fibrillation. Atrial fibrillation is an abnormal and irregular heartbeat that is usually caused by structural damage to the heart muscle or heart valves. When this cardiac arrhythmia is present, the heart beats erratically and blood does not flow smoothly. A complication that can occur from atrial fibrillation is the development of a blood clot within the chambers of the heart. Heart valves act as one-way doors in the heart, allowing blood to move from chamber to chamber and through various vessels within the heart and preventing blood from backing up in the chamber or vessel above it. Consequently, with this cardiac arrhythmia, when the heart beats, the clot can break loose from the heart and be passed along to the brain, causing a brain attack. It might be passed to other organs or extremities, causing an obstruction that prevents normal blood flow. This can cause necrosis or death of the organ or extremity in question due to the lack of oxygen and blood flow.

Many individuals with cardiovascular disease also have a proclivity to develop diabetes. When uncontrolled, diabetes adversely affects circulation. When diabetes is not adequately controlled due to diet, exercise, and adequate intrinsic or extrinsic insulin supply, the cells of the body become nutritionally compromised. Insulin is a naturally excreted hormone produced by the pancreas. Clients who are deficient in the production of insulin or who have other problems that prevent the insulin from attaching to the cells appropriately need to take insulin injections to compensate for this deficit. Extrinsic insulin supply is insulin that is administered to the client by means of injection or other methods. Intrinsic insulin supply is insulin that naturally occurs or is formed in the body. The main nutritional supplements for cell survival are blood and oxygen, which are the major components involved with circulation and cardiovascular status. When the circulation is compromised due to the complications of diabetes, adequate amounts of blood and oxygen are not delivered to the cells of the body. When the cells of the body are deprived of their nutrients, cellular death or necrosis can occur. This explains why many seeking medical assistance are often experiencing acute exacerbations of a chronic disease process. Therefore, the client is usually more debilitated and incapacitated before seeking medical assistance, necessitating more involved comprehensive and sustainable care. However, many who live with a chronic disease can remain relatively stable in that disease process while being maintained and sustained on specific medications and or treatments.

The *Healthy People 2010* goal 12, "Improve cardiovascular health and quality of life through prevention, detection, and treatment of risk factors; early identification and treatment of heart attacks and strokes; and prevention of recurrent cardiovascular events," was chosen as the goal to be assessed in this chapter. The reasons for this include the interrelationship of several disease processes of heart disease, stroke (brain attack), hypertension, diabetes, renal disease, and others in this category.

As has already been discussed in Chapter 1, the Ontario Needs Impact Based Model can help guide a community assessment project. The framework/model provides a point of reference for data collection. Concepts or elements within a theoretical framework or model can be transposed into categories for data collection, needs identification, and planning.

Figures 3-1 to 3-4 illustrate adaptations of the outcome-present state-test model, or OPT Model, of clinical reasoning (Pesut, 1999) for application in assessing community health and wellness. Although this model is specifically a nursing process model, it is adapted here to represent a model for a community assessment project. In any client group, a core identifier or common *present state* disease process can be distinguished within the target population. By *reasoning* what symptoms and disease processes are associated with the core, needs can be identified and determinations for *outcomes* and the necessary recommendations to meet the outcomes can be made.

The circle in the middle of Figure 3-1 represents the primary disease process of the present state of the targeted population. In essence, this is the point of reference for further data collection (demonstrated in Figures 3-2, 3-3, and 3-4). Cardiac disease, including contributory factors and ramifications, will be used as the point of reference.

These figures can be fully utilized as a model while conducting an assessment of physical health and wellness needs for aggregates of a target population. Consider a group of clients with cardiac disease in a free standing clinic. Clients in this category, with the present state of cardiac disease, will represent the core or the point of reference in Figure 3-1.

Figure 3-1 ▪ Heart Disease as a Point of Reference for Assessment

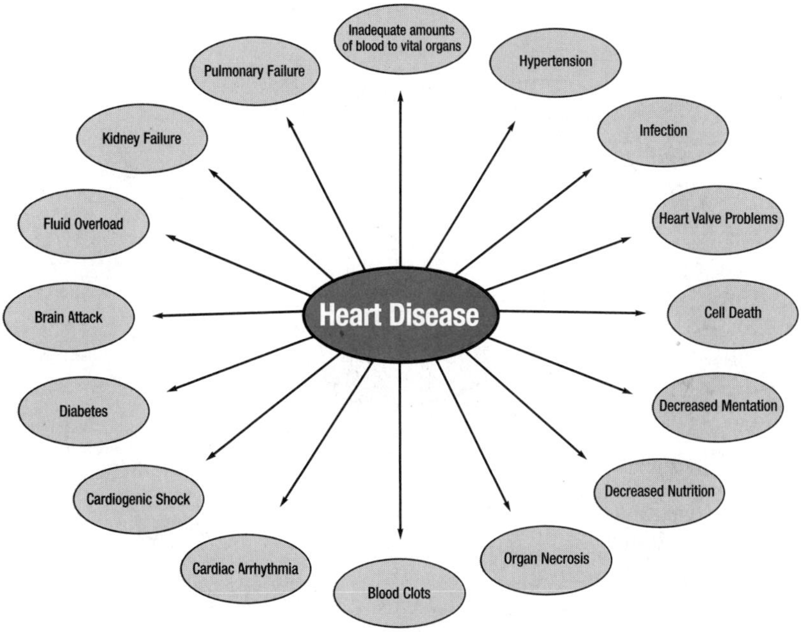

Adapted from Pesut, D., & Herman, J. (1999). *Clinical reasoning: The art and science of critical and creative thinking.* Clifton Park, NY: Delmar Learning.

To determine heart disease processes and the management needed for regulation and administration of care, Figures 3-2, 3-3, and 3-4 can be utilized. Figure 3-2 reveals the processes or elements that extend from the point of reference or present state of heart disease. These can further be transposed into other integrated categories for purposes of data collection, needs identification, and planning. By reasoning what symptoms and interrelated disease processes are associated with the present state of heart disease, outcomes can then be determined.

Each of the identified symptoms and associated disease processes will be represented in the outreaching circles visualized in Figure 3-2. The information presented in the outreaching circles manifests the complexity of heart disease.

A two-way vector is represented in this figure. Each spoke represents either a complication or associated potential disease process that is likely to be seen or diagnosed in clients who have heart disease and vice-versa. In essence, the problem or point of reference of the present state of heart disease has been defined. The problem of the present state of heart disease has been identified, and assessment and determination of outcomes

Figure 3-2 ▪ Relationship of Heart Disease to Other Disease Processes

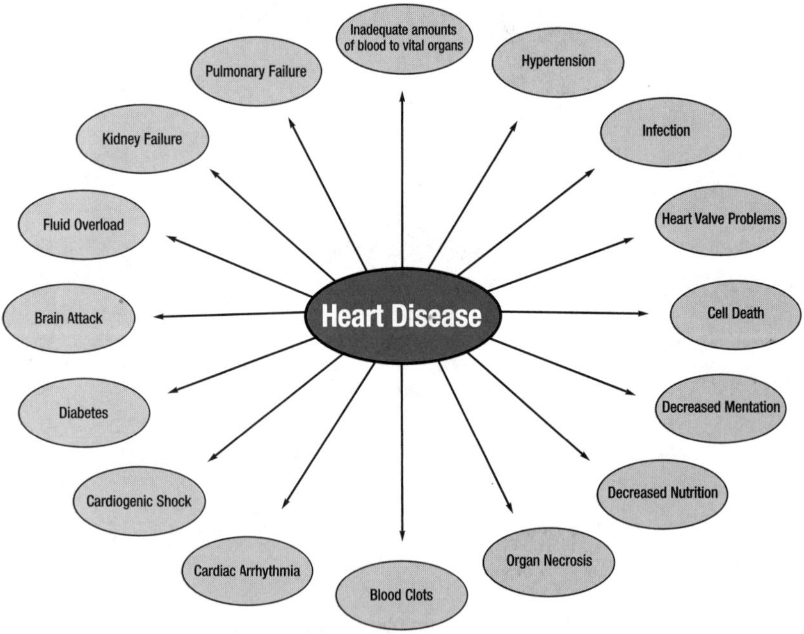

Adapted from Pesut, D., & Herman, J. (1999). *Clinical reasoning: The art and science of critical and creative thinking.* Clifton Park, NY: Delmar Learning.

associated with the problem are articulated by means of reasoning and defining the real and potential associated problems or complications.

All outreaching complications or associated potential disease processes identified in each circle of the spoke further distinguish populations of clients from which detailed information can be obtained for purposes of data collection, needs identification, and planning. These outreaching identifiers can also be used to identify clients who present with these recognized complications or associated potential disease processes as primary complaints. These clients can then be considered potential candidates for other associated, although not identified, primary health care needs.

Figure 3-3 can be utilized to reveal further extensions of the point of reference of the present state of heart disease. A projection of a complication of other associated symptoms or disease processes such as hypertension is used in this example. By means of reasoning, it can be deduced that not only can heart disease cause hypertension, but hypertension can also cause complications or associated potential disease processes that are likely to be seen or diagnosed in clients who have heart disease. Thus, outcomes can be determined based upon the findings.

Figure 3-3 ■ Interrelationship of Heart Disease and Other Disease Processes

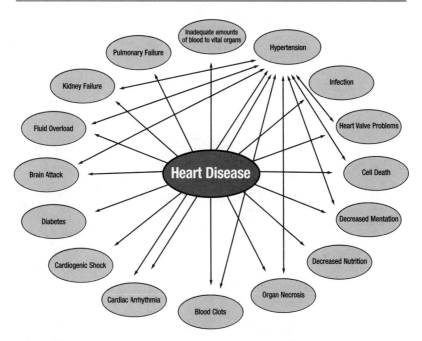

Adapted from Pesut, D., & Herman, J. (1999). *Clinical reasoning: The art and science of critical and creative thinking.* Clifton Park, NY: Delmar Learning.

Redundancy seems to be present, but in reality, a direct interrelationship and continuing and ongoing two-way vector of all these disease processes is evident. As identified in Figure 3-3, hypertension can be a direct correlate of heart valve problems. In critical situations, cellular death and organ necrosis can be manifested, with more specific complications of renal failure and fluid overload. With the presence of heart disease and hypertension, cardiac arrhythmias and blood clots are possible. Also, hypertension can be a direct corresponding complication of reduced mentation or brain attack due to the decreased amount of blood flow from the primary cause of the heart problem, from the potential complication of blood clots, or from any of the other direct interrelationships of symptoms and complications associated with hypertension.

Figure 3-4 takes the concept of the two-way vector one step further. Not only can the point of reference (heart disease) exhibit congruency with the outliers of the point of reference and the interrelationships between them; direct interrelationships are also manifested between the outliers themselves.

Figure 3-4 ■ The Compounding of Effects on Each Other and the Point of Reference

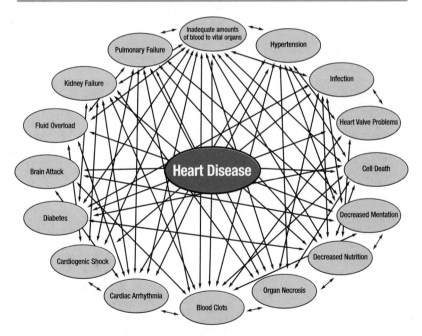

Adapted from Pesut, D., & Herman, J. (1999). *Clinical reasoning: The art and science of critical and creative thinking.* Clifton Park, NY: Delmar Learning.

These models visually demonstrate not only the problem or the identified present state, but also, by means of reasoning, can easily help to determine other information and outcomes that can be required for thorough data gathering as well as the management needed for regulation and administration of care for the targeted population under investigation. This data can lead to the comprehensive analysis and determination of outcomes of the information at hand.

Once the context of present state of the target population is identified, by means of reasoning, data can be assessed within the confines of the target population. Needs and outcomes can be identified and recommendations can be made.

In conclusion, to determine what information is required to adequately perform a community health and wellness needs assessment, the researcher must: (1) determine the objective, (2) establish and investigate the target population to be assessed, (3) assess the data, (4) analyze the data, and (5) make recommendations. Table 3-2 presents the rationale for each step.

Diabetes mellitus is a disease that is classified by high levels of glucose detected in the blood. This overabundance of glucose results from defective insulin secretion, insulin action, or both. There are four types of diabetes. Type 1 diabetes is also known as insulin-dependent diabetes mellitus (IDDM), or juvenile-onset diabetes. Type 2 diabetes is also known as non-insulin dependent diabetes mellitus (NIDDM), or adult-onset diabetes. Gestational diabetes develops in 2 percent to 5 percent of

TABLE 3-2 Rationale for Conducting a Needs Assessment in a Stepwise Fashion

FUNCTION	RATIONALE
Determine the objective.	The objective describes what you want the assessment to accomplish.
Establish and investigate the target population.	The target population consists of those who are affected by or who are at risk for the condition being assessed.
Assess data.	Data must be assessed from all possible domains.
Analyze data.	Analysis results in the identification of a need, or verifies that no such need exists.
Make recommendations.	Recommendations for action are based on findings and guided by current practices.

all pregnancies but disappears when a pregnancy is over. "Other types" of diabetes result from specific genetic syndromes, surgery, drugs, malnutrition, infections, and other illnesses (National Center for Chronic Disease Prevention and Health Promotion Diabetes Public Health Resource, 2001).

Step Three: Information Gathering

Once the objective for the assessment has been determined and the target population has been established, investigation and information gathering can begin. Information must be acquired and assessed from all possible domains. Information can be gathered in a number of different ways. With the advent of the Internet, information can be obtained by the mere click of a button on a keyboard. Information searches can be performed by means of conventional methods with the use of search engines. Data banks such as Cumulative Index to Nursing and Allied Health Literature (CINAHL), which is a data bank resource specific for nursing research information, can also be used. Another way to obtain information is to utilize the library. Contacting local and state Boards of Health can also provide a plethora of available data. National data banks of information from the Centers for Disease Control (CDC) can also help establish norms for specific client profiles. For purposes of this book and chapter, all of the above means of research were used and utilized.

In addition, the following goals and benchmarks from *Healthy People 2010* were chosen because they address the position of the client with a chronic disease who may have interrelated disease processes. This chapter also demonstrates the assessment of areas of functioning that contribute to overall physical wellness.

Goal Two: Arthritis

Goal 2 is "Improve illness and disability related to arthritis and other rheumatic conditions, osteoporosis, and chronic back conditions." There are nine objectives for goal 2 (Nardi, Sutherland, Tippy, Strupeck, et al., 2001, p. 21). These objectives measure range of motion, flexibility, the ability to function in the modes of daily living, pain management, increased access to treatment, and decreased hospitalizations. In essence, this goal relates to the definition and description of the needs assessment problem based upon the assumptions of normal Activities of Daily Living established by normal activity, mobility, and pain management. Examples of disease processes associated with this goal include arthritis and rheumatic conditions. For instance, in 1990, in one Midwestern state, 15 percent of non-institutionalized older persons reported a mobility limitation that made it difficult to go outside the home alone. Eleven percent reported a self-care limitation, which made it difficult to take care of their own personal needs (Teclaw, Gamache, Dorrell, Hile, Lewis, Starkey, Stemnock, & Thomas, 2001). For a client who has an underlying disease process with a mobility problem, incapacitation will be further pronounced due to the underlying circulatory deficit. Some other resources that can be used to gather data regarding this goal at the national or state level can be found at web searches on state statistics and emergency departments at local hospitals. Other information regarding arthritis can be found at the web site available at the time this book was written: http://www.wvhealth.wvu.edu/clinical/arthritis/abut.htm.

Goal Three: Cancer

Goal 3 is "Reduce the number of new cancer cases as well as the illness, disability, and death caused by cancer." There are nine objectives for this goal (Nardi, Sutherland, Tippy, Strupeck, et al., 2001, p. 22), which address the conjectures that a diagnosis of cancer has been made or can be made by means of primary health care preventative procedures. **Primary health care** is normally the entry point to the health care delivery system. The client is usually sick enough to realize that simple remedies are not resolving the problem. This can occur with the understanding and assumption that the health care delivery system is available and can be accessed by the client in need. Once the primary health care system has been accessed, the understanding is that secondary health care interventions and tertiary health care interventions will be provided. **Secondary health care** involves treatment of a disease process in the acute phase. This might include something as simple as taking prescribed medications to temporarily halt or eliminate the progression of a disease process. **Tertiary health care** addresses actions taken to limit the course of a disease process. An example might be a client undergoing coronary artery bypass graft surgery due to blockage of his or her coronary arteries.

Goal Four: Kidney Disease

Goal 4 is: "Reduce new cases of chronic kidney disease and its complications, disability, death, and economic costs." There are four objectives for this goal (Nardi, Sutherland, Tippy, Strupeck, et al., 2001, p. 24). As has already been discussed, chronic renal disease has a direct interrelationship with certain cardiac and other diseases. Objectives for goal 4 address issues of client diagnosis, compliance, and long-term treatment for this chronic disease. Other issues alluded to in this section also address the holistic approach in client support and care in relation to potential for kidney transplant and potential for post-donor organ failure. For instance, in 1999, the incidence rates for new cases of end stage renal disease (ESRD) in Indiana was 305 cases per million population. Also, in the same year, the incidence rates for new clients on dialysis in Indiana was 883 cases per million population. In addition, the primary diagnoses associated with these numbers of newly diagnosed ESRD clients were diabetes (739) followed by hypertension (429) (Kheirbek, 2000). Treatment for ESRD is federally funded. More information on a nationwide level can be obtained at the web site available at the time this book was written: http://www.cnn.com/ALLPOLITICS/resources/2000/pdf/budget.pdf.

Goal Five: Diabetes

Goal 5 is "Through prevention programs, reduce the disease and economic burden of diabetes and improve the quality of life for all persons who have or at risk for diabetes." This goal has 17 related objectives (Nardi, Sutherland, Tippy, Strupeck, et al., 2001, p. 25). Again, objectives for goal 5 relate to the interrelationship of diabetes with chronic cardiac and vascular problems. Issues not considered here also relate to potential loss of vision as well as potential for limb amputation due to damage of the microvessels in the vascular system. Microvessels are also called capillaries. Capillaries are the smallest vessels and allow for the exchange of waste products from the oxygenated blood to be carried through the veins and venules. Transportation continues through the blood to the arteries, which contain oxygenated blood. In the diabetic patient, if the vessels are compromised because of the lack of adequate circulation, the tissues that would normally receive the blood and oxygen supplied by the circulation will not be able to do so and will necrose or die because of the lack of nutrients or blood and oxygen. In 1998, diabetes was the third leading cause of deaths among Blacks between the ages of 55 and 64 (Teclaw, Gamache, Dorrell, Hile, Lewis, Starkey, Stemnock, & Thomas, 2001).

Goal Twelve: Cardiac Health

Goal 12 is "Improve cardiovascular health and quality of life through prevention, detection, and treatment of risk factors; early identification and treatment of heart attacks and strokes; and prevention of recurrent cardiovascular events." The common term for strokes is now brain attack.

This goal has 17 related objectives (Nardi, Sutherland, Tippy, Strupeck, et al., 2001, p. 37).

Objectives for goal 12 address issues of client education, compliance with treatment, medication, diet, and activity levels. Also included here are again the implications for multisystem disease processes. More information about this goal will be addressed later in this chapter.

Goal Nineteen: Healthy Diet and Weight

Goal 19 is "Promote health and reduce chronic disease associated with diet and weight." There are 17 objectives related to goal 19 (Nardi, Sutherland, Tippy, Strupeck, et al., 2001, pp. 50–51). Objectives for goal 19 are associated with overall physical wellness as well as potential complications of interrelated disease processes, especially diabetes.

Goal Twenty-One: Oral and Craniofacial Diseases

Goal 21 is "Prevent and control oral and craniofacial diseases, conditions, and injuries and improve access to related services." There are 15 objectives related to this goal (Nardi, Sutherland, Tippy, Strupeck, et al., 2001, p. 53).

Adequate dental and oral health is directly associated with appropriate nutritional status. Nutritional status is directly associated with an overall well-being of cellular health. Craniofacial diseases and injuries affect the ability to maintain appropriate nutritional status. In 1989, the average income of those age 65 and over was less than $15,000 (Annual Report to Congress, 2001). Again, income is directly related to adequate nutritional status.

Goal Twenty-Four: Respiratory Health

Goal 24 is "Promote respiratory health through better prevention, detection, treatment, and education." Nine objectives are associated with this goal (Nardi, Sutherland, Tippy, Strupeck, et al., 2001, p. 59). According to information found at http://www.cdc.gov/nceh/asthma/factsheets/asthma.htm, almost one-third of all inflicted with asthma are children. Nationally, the incidence of episode or attack of asthma within a 12-month period has increased. In 1998, an average of 14.5 people died each day from asthma. Since 1977, death rates from asthma for all age groups have risen; death rates from asthma have tripled in the past two decades. Incidence of asthma in Blacks is higher than Whites for all age groups (Pew Environmental Health Commission, 2000).

Chronic obstructive pulmonary disease is a common correlate to underlying cardiovascular disease and is related to cigarette smoking. The significant factors associated with the objectives for goal 24 are education and compliance of treatment for adults as well as children. Information about respiratory health can be obtained at http://www.cdc.gov/nceh/asthma/brochures/airpollution.htm. Information about the local statistics of respiratory diseases can be obtained through local state Boards of Health as well as facilities such as the local hospitals and school systems.

Goal Twenty-Eight: Vision and Hearing

Goal 28 is "Improve the visual and hearing health of the Nation through prevention, early detection, treatment, and rehabilitation." Fourteen objectives are related to this goal (Nardi, Sutherland, Tippy, Strupeck, et al., 2001, pp. 67–68). Objectives for goal 28 deal with availability of services to adults and children for purposes of vision screening, glaucoma testing, and noise prevention. In 1975, one-third of persons age 70 and older were reported to be hearing impaired (Kramarow, Lentzer, Rooks, Weeks, & Saydah, 1999).

Again, there is a direct interrelationship of blindness and diabetes as well as diabetes and cardiovascular disease. This further substantiates the interrelationship of disease processes. Information and statistics regarding visual and hearing health as well as social, epidemiological, and health-related issues can be found at http://www.cdc.gov/nchs/data/hus99cht.pdf.

Step Four: Analysis of the Information

Analysis of information in a health and wellness needs assessment can be linked to outcomes identified as the concept of illness behavior. **Illness behavior** occurs when a decision is made by the patient to seek medical care and what type of care to seek. The decision is usually based on the type and severity of symptoms experienced. Many sociological theories address the concept of illness behavior. One definition defines illness behavior as behavior beginning prior to the use of services which shapes decisions about whether to seek care and what type to help to solicit (Mechanic, 1992, in Matcha, 2001, p. 141). In 1965, Suchman's Stages of Illness Experience Model was developed and presented. Suchman's model addresses five stages, from symptom experience to recuperation.

Stage One is *Symptom Experience.* In this stage, there is an awareness of the existence of a medical problem. Symptoms are often benign and indicate no cause for concern. In Stage Two, *Assumption of the Sick Role,* acknowledgment of the sick role is validated by significant others of the person assuming that role. Symptoms are now obvious not only to the client, but also to the client's significant others. Suchman's *Assumption of the Sick Role* can be equated with the concept of primary health care in that the entry point to the health care delivery system actually begins here. The client is usually sick enough to realize that simple remedies are not resolving the problem.

In Stage Three, *Medical Care Contact,* the person assuming the sick role seeks professional assistance toward the attainment of an again healthy state. In reality, of course, this is dependent upon the availability and location of health care services to that person. Suchman's Stage Three, *Medical Care Contact,* equates with the secondary intervention process, in that treatment of a disease process occurs in the acute phase. The *Dependent Client Role,* Stage Four, allows the client to assume the sick role by becoming dependent on the recommendations and treatments of the physician or health care practitioner or provider. Tertiary intervention might be included in this phase, depending on the events taken to limit the course of a disease process.

Stage Five, *Recovery or Rehabilitation,* occurs when the client relinquishes the sick role and moves to a state of recovery and normal Activities of Daily Living. In this stage, the client with a chronic disease may have eliminated the acute exacerbation of the disease process but due to the fact that the disease is still present, will continue to remain in the classification of the client role even though he or she is deemed healthy at this point. In the present era of the aging population, the significance of this final stage is becoming continuously more profound (Matcha, 2001, pp. 141–143).

Suchman's Stages of Illness Experience Model can easily be assimilated to fit with the purposes and proposed outcomes of *Healthy People 2010.* Suchman's model addresses identification of the state of illness, entry into the health system, and proposed outcomes based on the acute or chronic state of the client. *Healthy People 2010* delineates targets of existing disease processes of a chronic nature, identified needs, and recommendations. Both *Healthy People 2010* and Suchman's model indirectly yet poignantly address the present situation of an aging society with chronic health problems associated with frequent episodes of limited access to health care means and modalities.

Disparities in the levels of availability and access to health care appear to be a common theme in today's society. Continuous biomedical achievements seem to want to prolong life at any cost (Mason & Leavitt, 1998). Yet, the reality in most situations is that when services are available, many times what takes place is the adoption of a community service model. This model utilizes cost cutting values, giving the client just the right amount of services for just as long as he or she needs it (Curtain, 2001). An example of this is our present-day model of managed care and the health maintenance organization (HMO). Within the context of these two entities, cost cutting measures are implemented by means of mandated limited time spent with clients. The use of a group of physicians for the clients enrolled in the HMO further enhances the utilization of available services to the client, but decreases the continuity of care for the client usually seen by one specific physician. Limited services available under the health care plan further exacerbate the problem (Matcha, 2001, pp. 49, 251). It appears that healthy individuals and those who are not sick or have chronic diseases are encouraged to enroll in Medicare HMOs as HMOs seem to cater to health prevention and health maintenance rather than to those with chronic health problems (Neumann, Maibach, Dusenbury et al., 1998; Annual Report to Congress, 1996; Portell, Cocotas, Parales et al., 1996, in Harrington & Estes, 2001, p. 227). In essence, the total number of clients cared for under capitation will usually determine reimbursement by insurance and third-party payers. Therefore, profits obtained by health care providers are more fully realized by the maintenance of a caseload of young and healthy clients who will, in essence, remain in that state with the utilization of ongoing health prevention and health maintenance regimens.

CONSTRUCTING A NEEDS ASSESSMENT TOOL

Needs are usually based on findings from a survey, appraisal, evaluation, critique, or assessment. The use and implementation of a health assessment needs tool is one such method of determining what the needs are in a given population of clients. When examining the results of the needs assessment tool of a group of clients with common characteristics, it stands to reason that results would reveal common characteristics. An example would be clients who are older and have a primary diagnosis of cardiovascular problems. Findings would most likely reveal the interrelationships of the already discussed and demonstrated disease processes as will be further examined below.

Healthy People 2010 objectives focus on symptom experience as defined in Suchman's Stages of Illness Experience Model and can be linked to *Healthy People 2010* goal 12: "Improve cardiovascular health and quality of life through prevention, detection, and treatment of risk factors; early identification and treatment of heart attacks and strokes; and prevention of recurrent cardiovascular events." In the stage of symptom experience,

TABLE 3-3 Example: Needs Assessment Physical Health and Wellness *continued*

GOAL TWELVE: Improve cardiovascular health and quality of life through prevention, detection and treatment of risk factors; early identification and treatment of heart attacks and strokes; and prevention of recurrent cardiovascular events

HP 2010 OBJECTIVES	TARGET	DATA ASSESSED	NEED	RECOMMENDATIONS
1. Reduce coronary heart disease deaths	To 166 deaths per 100,000 population	In 1997, the five leading causes of death in Gary were: heart disease (343 cases), malignant neoplasms (269 cases); homicide (89 cases); cerebrovascular disease (80 cases) and diabetes mellitus (532 cases) (Indiana State, 1998).	X	Develop a regional health and wellness center, affiliated with area hospitals, to meet primary health needs of the underserved.
2. Increase proportion of adults > 20 who are aware of the early warning symptoms of a heart attack and the importance of accessing rapid emergency care by calling 911	Total coverage	In 1996, the number of Indiana residents who were discharged from hospitals in the state for these cardiac-related diagnoses were: 9,572; chestpain, 8,886; (Indiana Hospital Consumer Guide, 1996).	X	The health and wellness center will include a health education program and outreach efforts to advise the primary health are services offered by the center.
3. Increase proportion of eligible clients with heart attacks who receive artery-opening therapy	Within an hour of symptom onset	In 1996, the number of Indiana residents who were discharged from hospitals in the state for these cardiac-related diagnoses	X	Develop a regional health and wellness center, affiliated with area hospitals, to meet primary health needs of the underserved while

continues

TABLE 3-3 Example: Needs Assessment Physical Health and Wellness *continued*

HP 2010 OBJECTIVES	TARGET	DATA ASSESSED	NEED	RECOMMENDATIONS
		were: percutaneous cardiovascular procedures, 9,572; other vascular procedures, 4,385; coronary bypass with cardiac catheterization, 4,190; percutaneous cardiovascular procedures with acute myocardial infarction, 3,885 (Indiana Hospital Consumer Guide, 1996).		educating the public by means of health education programs through outreach efforts which advertise the primary health care services offered by the center. Bring the health education programs to the public in affiliation with schools, churches, community centers, senior high rise building etc. Study the effectiveness of the Emergency Care Systems (EMS) in NW Indiana.
4. Increase proportion of adults > 20 who call 911 and administer CPR when they witness an out-of-hospital cardiac arrest	Total coverage	Heart disease was the leading cause of death (16,483 cases) in Indiana (Center for Disease Control, 2000). In Lake county, deaths from major cardiovascular disease totaled 1,858; deaths from disease for the heart were 1,452; deaths from ischemic heart disease were 989; deaths from acute myocardial infarction were	X	Bring health education programs to the public in affiliation with schools, churches, community centers, senior high rise building etc. Study the effectiveness of the Emergency Care Systems (EMS) in NW Indiana.

continues

350; deaths from old myocardial infarction and related cardiac disease were 635; deaths from other forms of heart disease were 432; deaths from hypertension with or without renal disease were 29; deaths from cerebrovascular diseases were 301 (Indiana State, 1998).

In Porter county, deaths from major cardiovascular disease totaled 427; deaths from disease of the heart were 309; deaths from ischemic heart disease were 187; deaths from acute myocardial infarction were 71; deaths from old myocardial infarction and related cardiac disease were 116; deaths from other forms of heart disease were 115; deaths from hypertension with or without renal disease were 10; deaths from cerebrovascular diseases were 80 (Indiana State, 1998).

TABLE 3-3   Example: Needs Assessment Physical Health and Wellness   *continued*

HP 2010 OBJECTIVES	TARGET	DATA ASSESSED	NEED	RECOMMENDATIONS
		In LaPorte county, deaths from major cardiovascular disease totaled 414; deaths from disease of the heart were 326; deaths from ischemic heart disease were 204; deaths from acute myocardial infarction were 110; deaths from old myocardial infarction and related cardiac disease were 92; deaths from other forms of heart disease were 104; deaths from hypertension with or without renal disease were 5; deaths from cerebrovascular diseases were 57 (Indiana State, 1998).		
5. Increase the proportion of persons with witnessed out-of-hospital cardiac arrest who are eligible and receive therapeutic shock within 6 minutes after collapse recognition	Total coverage	In 1997, several of the leading causes of death in Gary were: heart disease (343 cases), cerebrovascular disease (80 cases) and diabetes mellitus (532 cases) (Indiana State, 1998).	X	Study the effectiveness of the Emergency Care Systems (EMS) in NW Indiana. Develop a regional health and wellness center, affiliated with area hospitals, to meet primary health needs of the underserved while educating

the public by means of health education programs through outreach efforts which advertise the primary health care services offered by the center.

6. Reduce hospitalizations of older adults with heart failure as the principal diagnosis.	Total coverage	In 1996, the number of Indiana residents who were discharged from hospitals in the state for these cardiac-related diagnoses were: 21,656 for heart failure and shock; (Indiana Hospital Consumer Guide, 1996). In 1999, cardiology-related diagnoses, including heart failure, ranked second for all inclient DRG's at Methodist Hospitals (C. Biancardi, Methodist Hospitals, personal communication, Oct. 23, 2000).	X	Bring health education programs to the public in affiliation with schools, churches, community centers, senior high rise building etc. Design and fund an accessible transportation plan to the health and wellness center for the underserved.
7. Reduce stroke deaths	To 48 deaths per 100,00 population	In 1996, the number of Indiana residents who were discharged from hospitals in the state for these cardiac-related diagnoses were: specific cerebrovascular disorders except transient	X	Bring health education programs to the public in affiliation with schools, churches, community centers, senior high rise building etc. Study the effectiveness of the Emergency Care Systems (EMS)

continues

TABLE 3-3 Example: Needs Assessment Physical Health and Wellness *continued*

HP 2010 OBJECTIVES	TARGET	DATA ASSESSED	NEED	RECOMMENDATIONS
		ischemic attacks, 11,536; (Indiana Hospital Consumer Guide, 1996). In 1997, several leading causes of death in Gary were: heart disease (343 cases), cerebrovascular disease (80 cases) and diabetes mellitus (532 cases) (Indiana State, 1998).		in NW Indiana.
8. Increase proportion of adults who are aware of the early warning symptoms and signs of stroke	Total coverage	In Lake county, deaths from major cardiovascular disease totaled 1,858; deaths from disease for the heart were 1,452; deaths from ischemic heart disease were 989; deaths from acute myocardial infarction were 350; deaths from old myocardial infarction and related cardiac disease were 635; deaths from other forms of heart disease were 432; deaths from hypertension with or without renal disease were 29; deaths from	X	Develop a regional health and wellness center, affiliated with area hospitals, to meet primary health needs of the underserved while educating the public by means of health education programs through outreach efforts which advertise the primary health care services offered by the center. Bring health education programs to the public in affiliation with schools, churches, community centers, senior high rise building etc.

continues

cerebrovascular diseases were 301 (Indiana State, 1998).

In Porter county, deaths from major cardiovascular disease totaled 427; deaths from disease of the heart were 309; deaths from ischemic heart disease were 187; deaths from acute myocardial infarction were 71; deaths from old myocardial infarction and related cardiac disease were 116; deaths from other forms of heart disease were 115; deaths from hypertension with or without renal disease were 10; deaths from cerebrovascular diseases were 80 (Indiana State, 1998).

In LaPorte county, deaths from major cardiovascular disease totaled 414; deaths from disease of the heart were 326; deaths from ischemic heart disease were 204; deaths from acute myocardial infarction were 110; deaths from old myocardial infarction

TABLE 3-3 Example: Needs Assessment Physical Health and Wellness *continued*

HP 2010 OBJECTIVES	TARGET	DATA ASSESSED	NEED	RECOMMENDATIONS
		and related cardiac disease were 92; deaths from other forms of heart disease were 104; deaths from hypertension with or without renal disease were 5; deaths from cerebrovascular diseases were 57 (Indiana State, 1998).		
9. Reduce the proportion of adults with high blood pressure	To 16%	29.8% of NWI area adults have been diagnosed with high blood pressure; 20.5% have been told that their blood cholesterol levels were too high (PRC Community Health Assessment, 1996).	X	Bring health education programs to the public in affiliation with schools, churches, community centers, senior high rise building etc. Design and fund an accessible transportation plan to the health and wellness center for the underserved.
10. Increase proportion of adults with high blood pressure whose blood pressure is under control	To 50%	In Lake county, deaths from major cardiovascular disease totaled 1,858; deaths from disease for the heart were 1,452; deaths from ischemic heart disease were 989; deaths from acute myocardial infarction were	X	Design and fund an accessible transportation plan to the health and wellness center for the underserved.

350; deaths from old myocardial infarction and related cardiac disease were 635; deaths from other forms of heart disease were 432; deaths from hypertension with or without renal disease were 29; deaths from cerebrovascular diseases were 301 (Indiana State, 1998).

In Porter county, deaths from major cardiovascular disease totaled 427; deaths from disease of the heart were 309; deaths from ischemic heart disease were 187; deaths from acute myocardial infarction were 71; deaths from old myocardial infarction and related cardiac disease were 116; deaths from other forms of heart disease were 115; deaths from hypertension with or without renal disease were 10; deaths from cerebrovascular diseases were 80 (Indiana State, 1998).

continues

TABLE 3-3 Example: Needs Assessment Physical Health and Wellness *continued*

HP 2010 OBJECTIVES	TARGET	DATA ASSESSED	NEED	RECOMMENDATIONS
		In LaPorte county, deaths from major cardiovascular disease totaled 414; deaths from disease of the heart were 326; deaths from ischemic heart disease were 204 ; deaths from acute myocardial infarction were 110; deaths from old myocardial infarction and related cardiac disease were 92; deaths from other forms of heart disease were 104; deaths from hypertension with or without renal disease were 5; deaths from cerebrovascular diseases were 57 (Indiana State, 1998).		
11. Increase proportion of adults with high blood pressure who are taking action (i.e.: losing weight, increasing physical activity, and reducing sodium intake), to help	To 95%	In 1998, 56% of Indiana residents reported having a sedentary lifestyle on the national Behavior Risk Factor Surveillance System (BRFSS). (Indiana Health Behavior, 1998).	X	Develop a regional health and wellness center, affiliated with area hospitals, to meet primary health needs of the underserved while educating the public by means of health education programs through outreach efforts which advertise the primary

Objective	Target	Status		Strategies
control their blood pressure.				health care services offered by the center. Bring health education programs to the public in affiliation with schools, churches, community centers, senior high rise building etc.
12. Increase proportion of adults who have had their blood pressure measured within the preceding 2 years and can state whether their blood pressure was normal or high.	To 95%	In 1997, 6.9% of Indiana adults > 18 years did not have their blood pressure checked for the two years preceding (National Center for Chronic Disease Prevention & Health Promotion, 2000).	X	Develop a regional health and wellness center, affiliated with area hospitals, to meet primary health needs of the underserved while educating the public by means of health education programs through outreach efforts which advertise the primary health care services offered by the center. Bring health education programs to the public in affiliation with schools, churches, community centers, senior high rise building etc.
13. Reduce the mean of total cholesterol levels among adults	To 199 mg/dL	29.8% of NWI area adults have been diagnosed with high blood pressure; 20.5% have been told that their blood cholesterol levels were too high (PRC Community Health Assessment, 1996).	X	Develop a regional health and wellness center, affiliated with area hospitals, to meet primary health needs of the underserved while educating the public by means of health education programs through outreach

continues

TABLE 3-3 Example: Needs Assessment Physical Health and Wellness *continued*

HP 2010 OBJECTIVES	TARGET	DATA ASSESSED	NEED	RECOMMENDATIONS
				efforts which advertise the primary health care services offered by the center. Bring health education programs to the public in affiliation with schools, churches, community centers, senior high rise building etc.
14. Reduce proportion of adults with high total blood cholesterol levels	To 17%	29.8% of NWI area adults have been diagnosed with high blood pressure; 20.5% have been told that their blood cholesterol levels were too high (PRC Community Health Assessment, 1996).	X	Develop a regional health and wellness center, affiliated with area hospitals, to meet primary health needs of the underserved while educating the public by means of health education programs through outreach efforts which advertise the primary health care services offered by the center. Bring health education programs to the public in affiliation with schools, churches, community centers, senior high rise building etc.
15. Increase proportion of adults who have had their	To 80%	29.8% of NWI area adults have been diagnosed with high blood	X	Develop a regional health and wellness center, affiliated with area hos-

Objective		Data		Strategies
blood cholesterol checked within the preceding 5 years		pressure; 20.5% have been told that their blood cholesterol levels were too high (PRC Community Health Assessment, 1996).		pitals, to meet primary health needs of the underserved while educating the public by means of health education programs through outreach efforts which advertise the primary health care services offered by the center. Bring health education programs to the public in affiliation with schools, churches, community centers, senior high rise building etc.
16. Increase proportion of persons with coronary heart disease who have had their LDL-cholesterol level treated	To a goal of less than or equal to 100 mg/dL. **	29.8% of NWI area adults have been diagnosed with high blood pressure; 20.5% have been told that their blood cholesterol levels were too high (PRC Community Health Assessment, 1996).	X	Develop a regional health and wellness center, affiliated with area hospitals, to meet primary health needs of the underserved while educating the public by means of health education programs through outreach efforts which advertise the primary health care services offered by the center. Bring health education programs to the public in affiliation with schools, churches, community centers, senior high rise building etc.

**Specific Data not available

there is an awareness of an existence of a medical problem. An example might be a client experiencing chest pain and left arm weakness. Both are symptoms of a heart attack. If the client is informed and has an appreciation of the health problem, then when symptoms occur, assumption of the sick role and entry to the health care system can conceivably occur sooner and the client will spend a shorter time in that role.

Targets for improved health can be met if the assumption of the sick role is validated and occurs immediately upon acknowledgment of symptom experience. This means that if the client is knowledgeable of symptoms, possibly constituting a disease process, and assumes the sick role with validation of positive symptom identification, then improved targets can be met based specifically on client knowledge alone. Data assessed can be obtained through a secondary analysis of records. Data assessed, such as the data that was assessed in the needs assessment tool presented here, can also be obtained more quickly and efficiently if adequate medical care contact is available to the client. A medical care contact can be a primary care health physician, a free standing clinic, a nurse practitioner, attendance at a health fair, or blood pressure and other health screenings, just to name a few. Identified needs can help to lessen the time frame the individual remains in the dependent client role. Recommendations for recovery or rehabilitation can be equated to the objectives of *Healthy People 2010,* which are grounded on the four enabling goals and pertain to promoting healthful behaviors, protecting health, achieving access to quality health care, and strengthening community. The actions involved in a community assessment of health and wellness needs are outlined and summarized in Table 3-4.

 KEY POINTS

◆ The health status of a person directly parallels quality of life and the availability of health care services.

◆ The nine goals of *Healthy People 2010* address the assessment and functioning of overall physical health and wellness and demonstrate an interrelationship of chronic disease processes.

◆ For the client with a chronic multisystem disease process, such as the cardiac client, well-being seems to be associated with stability of the disease process.

◆ To determine what information is required to adequately perform a community health and wellness needs assessment, the researcher must: (1) determine the objective, (2) establish and investigate the

continues on p. 106

TABLE 3-4 Application of the Community Health and Wellness Assessment Processes

APPLICATION OF THE COMMUNITY HEALTH AND WELLNESS ASSESSMENT PROCESS	USE OF PRIMARY AND SECONDARY DATA RESOURCES
Before Beginning	The need of the current status of health coverage is visited and the need for coverage for all is implied.
Step One	Examines the concept of health and well-being from the standpoint of the World Health Organization and the nursing profession.
Step Two	Discusses an example of the interrelationship of disease processes from the standpoint of the cardiovascular client.
Step Three	Exhibits the nine goals of *Healthy People 2010* and discusses resources for further knowledge of each.
Step Four	Discusses Suchman's Stages of Illness Experience Model as it relates to the purposes and proposed outcomes of *Healthy People 2010*.
Targets or Benchmarks	Indicates desired results: Examples include those listed in Goal Twelve, Objective 1, *Reduce coronary heart disease deaths* with a target of *to 166 deaths per 100,000 population*.
Data Assessed	Reveals the findings of the target of the community that was assessed. In this example, one of the five leading causes of death in Gary in 1997 was heart disease.
Identified Need	Reveals issues and problems that are prevalent in the targeted community. In this example, a recommendation was made to develop a regional health and wellness center, affiliated with area hospitals, to meet primary health needs of the underserved. The development of such a center will not only provide needed services, but will more easily validate *Symptom Experience* to allow for a more rapid assumption of the sick role thus improving recommended targets.
Recommendations	Are based on social norms and expectations that guide present and future health services. Availability and access to health care and services are the key roles to the fulfillment and success of the cited and suggested recommendations.

KEY POINTS (*continued*)
> target population to be assessed, (3) assess the data, (4) analyze the data, (5) make recommendations.

◆ Once the target population has been established, investigation can begin; information can be acquired in a number of different ways.

◆ Primary health care is normally the entry point to the health care delivery system.

◆ Secondary health care involves treatment of a disease process in the acute phase.

◆ Tertiary health care addresses actions taken to limit the course of a disease process.

◆ Analysis of information can be linked to outcomes identified as the concept of illness behavior, which is made by the client to determine whether to seek medical care and what type of care to seek.

◆ Suchman's Stages of Illness Experience Model addresses five stages from symptom experience to recuperation: symptom experience, assumption of the sick role, medical care contact, dependent client role, and recovery or rehabilitation.

◆ *Healthy People 2010* objectives focus on symptom experience as defined in Suchman's Stages of Illness Experience Model and can be linked to *Healthy People 2010* goals.

 REFERENCES

American Academy of Audiology. (2000). *Status of hearing screening in each state.* Retrieved November 24, 2001, from http://www.infanthearing.org/states/indiana.html.

Annual Report to Congress. *Physician's Payment Review Commission.* (2001). Sudbury, MA. In Harrington, C., & Estes, C. (2001) *Health policy: Crisis and reform in the U.S. health care delivery system* (3rd. ed., p. 227). MA: Jones and Bartlett Publishers Research Center. Page updated September 1999 with 1998 population estimates. Retrieved November 24, 2001, from http://www.ibrc.indiana.edu/Population/older_profile.htm.

Arthritis: About Arthritis and Other Rheumatic Diseases. (2001). West Virginia Health Page. Retrieved November 24, 2001, from http://www.wvhealth.wvu.edu/clinical/arthritis/abut.htm.

Census Bureau, Employee Benefits Research Institute. (2000). In *Physicians for a National Health Program Newsletter* (2001). p. 3.

Centers for Disease Control. (2000). *DATA 2010: The Healthy People Database.* Retrieved November 24, 2001, from http://wonder.cdc.gov/nios.shtml.

CDC's Asthma Prevention Program. (2001). Retrieved November 24, 2001, from http://www.cdc.gov/nceh/asthma/factsheets/asthma.htm.

CHIP—Children's Health Insurance Program. (1997). Retrieved November 15, 2001, from http://www.in.gov/fssa/programs/chip/index.html.

Curtin, L. (2001). Healing the health care system. *Curtin Calls*. Metier Publications.

Data Update. (2001). Uninsured and underinsured. *Physicians for a National Health Program Newsletter.*

Division of Adult and Community Health, National Center for Chronic Disease Prevention and Health Promotion, Centers for Disease Control and Prevention, *Behavioral risk factor surveillance system* Online Prevalence Data, 1995–1998.

Donahue, J. M., & McGuire, M. B. (1995). The political economy of responsibility in health and illness. *Social Sciences in Medicine, 1* (40), 47–53. In Matcha, D. (2000). *Medical sociology.* Boston, MA: Allyn & Bacon.

Fiscal Year 2000 Budget. (2002). Budget of the United States Government. Retrieved November 24, 2001, from http://www.cnn.com/ALLPOLITICS/resources/2000/pdf/budget.pdf.

Gallo, J., Fulmer, T., Paveze, G. et al. (2000). *Handbook of geriatric assessment.* Gaithersburg, MD. Aspen Publication.

Harrington, C., & Estes, C. (2001). *Health policy: Crisis and reform in the U.S. health care delivery system* (3rd ed., p. 3). Sudbury, MA: Jones and Bartlett Publishers.

Health, United States 1999, Health and Aging Chartbook. Department of Health and Human Services. Retrieved November 24, 2001, from http://www.cdc.gov/nchs/data/hus99cht.pdf.

Healthy People 2000: Priority Areas and Area Resources. Retrieved November 15, 2001, from http://odphp.osophs.dhhs.gov/pubs/hp2000/prior.htm.

Himmelstein, D., Woolhandler, S. & Hellender, I. (2001). *Bleeding the patient: The consequences of corporate health care.* Monroe, ME: Common Courage Press.

Kheirbek, A. (2000). Personal interview, December 5, 2001. Information Retrieved in 1999 from http://www.therenalnetwork.org/.

Kramarow, E., Lentzer, H., Rooks, R., Weeks, J., & Saydah, S. (1999). *Health and aging chartbook.* Hyattsville, MD: National Center for Health Statistics.

Leading Indicators for Healthy People 2010. (1998). *First interim report.* Retrieved November 24, 2001, from http://www.nap.edu/html/healthy/.

Mason, D. & Leavitt, J. (1998). *Policy and politics in nursing and health care.* (3rd ed.). Philadelphia: Saunders.

Matcha, D. (2000). *Medical sociology.* Boston: Allyn and Bacon.

Mechanic, D. (1992). Health and illness behavior and patient-practitioner relationships. In Matcha, D. (2000). *Medical sociology.* Boston, MA: Allyn and Bacon.

Nardi, D., Sutherland, T., Tippy, F., Strupeck, D. et al. (2001). Needs assessment of the health and wellbeing of the Northwest Indiana region. Unpublished manuscript. Indiana University Northwest Shared Vision Research and Service Task Forces.

National Center for Chronic Disease Prevention & Health Promotion. (2000). *Behavioral risk factor surveillance system. BRFFS prevalence data*: Retrieved November 24, 2001, from http://www2.cdc.gov/nccdphp/brffs/index.asp.

National Center for Chronic Disease Prevention and Health Promotion Diabetes Public Health Resource. Retrieved November 14, 2001, from http://www.cdc.gov/diabetes/pubs/facts98.htm#types.

National Center for Environmental Health. (2001). *Asthma.* Retrieved November 24, 2001, from http://www.cdc.gov/nceh/asthma/brochures/airpollution.htm.

National Institute of Diabetes and Digestive and Kidney Disease. (2001). National Institute of Health. Retrieved November 24, 2001, from http://www.niddk.nih.gov/.

Neuman, P., Maibach, E., Dusenbury, K. et al. (1998). Marketing HMO's to Medicare beneficiaries: Do Medicare HMO's target healthy seniors? *Health Affairs (Millwood), 17,* 132–139.

Ottawa Charter for Health Promotion. (1986). Geneva: WHO. Retrieved November 24, 2001, from http://www.helsetilsynet.no/trykksak/fremmdok/glossary.htm.

Pesut, D., & Herman, J. (1999). Clinical reasoning: The art and science of critical and creative thinking. Clifton Park, NY: Delmar Learning.

Pew Environmental Health Commission. (2000). Attack asthma: Why America needs a public health defense system to battle environmental threats. Retrieved November 24, 2001, from http://pewenvirohealth.jhsph.edu/html/splash/text.html.

Physicians for a National Health Program: PNHP. (2000, September). PHNP newsletter, Chicago, IL: author.

Porell, F., Cocotas, C., Perelas, P., et al. (1992). Factors associated with disenrollment from Medicare HMO's: Finding from a survey of disenrollees. Report presented at a meeting at the Health Care Financing Administration, July 1992, for the Health Policy Research Consortium of Brandeis University.

Shortell, S., & Kaluzny, A. (2000). *Health care management: Organization design and behavior* (4th ed.). Clifton Park, NY: Delmar Learning.

Sultz, H., & Young, K. (2001). Health USA: Understanding its organization and delivery (3rd ed.). Aspen.

Teclaw, R., Gamache, R., Dorrell, S., Hile, W., Lewis, J., Starkey, M., Stemnock, L., & Thomas, C. (2001, May). *Indiana mortality report: State, county, and city data 1999.* Indianapolis: Indiana State Department of Health

United States Census 2000. Stats Indiana. Retrieved November 25, 2001 from http://www.shttp://www.stats.indiana.edu/c2k/c2kframe.htmltats.indiana.edu/c2k/c2kframe.html.

World Health Organization. (2001). *Definition of health. About WHO.* Retrieved November 24, 2001, from www.who.int/aboutwho/en/definition.html.

Chapter

4

ASSESSING
MENTAL HEALTH
AND WELLNESS

Susan Siwinski-Hebel

 LEARNING OBJECTIVES

At the conclusion of this chapter, the reader will be able to:

- ◆ Differentiate between mental health and mental illness.
- ◆ Explore the historical, social, and political implications that impact conducting a mental health and wellness needs assessment.
- ◆ Describe the steps of conducting a mental health and wellness needs assessment.
- ◆ Use *Healthy People 2010* goals and benchmarks as a framework for beginning examination of a community's mental health and wellness.
- ◆ Consider unique applications of community-specific data for data identification, gathering, and analysis.

KEY TERMS

Catchment area

Community mental health centers

Community support system (CSS)

Deinstitutionalization

Key stakeholders

Mental disorder

Mental health

Mental health services

Mental illness

Parity

Resilience

Serious mental illness (SMI)

There are many variables to consider when conducting an assessment of a community's needs. Conducting a mental health and wellness assessment for a community can be a daunting task with many factors to take into consideration. As in other chapters of this process guidebook, this chapter provides a comprehensive introduction to the current issues impacting the status of community mental health and wellness, the application of the assessment process, and resources that optimize efficiencies in cost and time. Whether the reader is an individual who is part of a public or private institution that perceives an existing need within the setting, but doesn't know how to substantiate his or her intuitive insights; a member of a team that has been given the task of writing a proposal addressing specific needs related to the promotion of mental health, prevention of mental illness, or management of existing mental disorders; or part of a consumer-based advocacy group focused on substantiating a need and achieving change, this chapter will provide a thorough application of the practice model and introduction to resources that will enhance the process of completing a thorough needs assessment.

Economic constraints have generated competition for funding among health care systems and limitations in delivery of health care services. Consequently, succinct communication of need as well as relevance of data that substantiates submitted requests is mandatory in securing funds. Tangible data becomes crucial in the identification of definitive needs. Secondary analysis of existing data guides the reader in considering data sets and resources that may provide beneficial information in validating needs. Data corresponding to four *Healthy People 2010* goals and related objectives are combined in this chapter and explored in their relationship to overall mental well-being in the United States. References for data are linked to each of the four goals presented. Next, the Ontario Needs Impact Based Model is applied to *Healthy People 2010* goal: "Improve mental health and access to appropriate, quality mental health services through improvements in mental health status, treatment expansion, and state activities to demonstrate relationship and findings for a targeted community population." Table 4-3 highlights the data and provides an example of assessing and analyzing it. Discussion and recommendations are also presented based on the findings and offer guidance for the planning of interventions for a specified community.

MENTAL HEALTH AND WELL-BEING: THE WHOLE IS LARGER THAN THE PARTS

The wholeness of a community needs assessment requires exploration of **mental health,** a state of being, defined by each individual according to actual or perceived satisfaction with his or her level of psychological functioning or according to prevailing or influencing sociocultural standards and well-being. Just as the literature in psychology and health care has taught that an individual cannot be assessed and treated by separating mind and body, the same applies to the overall mental health of a community. All the individuals who comprise a community wield influence upon that community's mental health and well-being. In addition, the awareness of a community's well-being can be broadened through an understanding of how its constituents interact with the prominent community systems. As a whole, these interactions establish a basis for the identity of the community. As mentioned in an earlier chapter of this book, the needs assessment should be approached from a holistic point of view. The concept of holism is very important in this chapter in that it is essential that the reader accept that a definite connection exists among the physical, psychological, spiritual, social, environmental, and economic realms of an individual's life in the United States and recognize that these factors impact the experience of health. Likewise, in conducting an assessment of the mental health and well-being of a community, the same premise must be incorporated as one assesses need.

Before additional examination of this area of need, a clear differentiation must be made between mental health and **mental illness.** The term "mental illness," a general term, is often used as a collective reference to any diagnosable **mental disorder.** Mental disorders are difficult to define succinctly. A disorder is comprised of a myriad of complex signs and symptoms that are interpreted based on varied levels of abstraction and psychological concepts. Clinical definitions represent disorders as clinically significant behavioral or psychological syndromes or patterns. Mental health is altered in the changes that occur to three primary factors: mood, behavior, and thought. Each factor can materialize as a separate alteration or in various combinations. The disorder may be perceived by the affected individual and associated with distress, disability, suffering, death, pain, or losses of freedom. Conversely, an individual may not have full awareness, understanding, or insight into a developing health problem. Disorders can occur in males or females of any age, race, or ethnic group. The etiologies, attributed to the development of disorders, have been correlated with positive family histories, genetics, and behavioral, biological, environmental, or social factors that occur independently or in combination (American Psychiatric Association [APA], 1994). Taking a thoughtful look at the World Health Organization (WHO) definition of health, it is understood that mental health in and of itself is not just the absence of a disease process. "Mental health is a state of well-being in which the individual realizes his or her own abilities, can cope with the normal stresses of life, can work productively and fruitfully, and is able to make a contribution to his or her community" (World Health Organization, 1999).

In the course of assessing the relative states of mental health and mental illness within a community, visualizing movement in wellness along a continuum is useful. The presence of mental wellness is influenced by the disposition of contributing variables. Movement along the continuum is the net total resulting from the influence of external and internal variables. This net result is the sum of all the variables' potential energy. Energy from the variables, positive as well as negative, exerts a force and crosses the dynamic boundary of community. The positive or negative nature of the sum energies generates a potential movement toward health or illness for a community at any point in time (see Figure 4-1).

Just as an individual moves back and forth along the continuum at any given time in response to multiple factors exerting some sort of force in his or her life, a community may also demonstrate similar movements.

A movement can occur within any segment of the community and is influenced by the variables impacting it at any point in time in its existence. An example of a community constituent, an external variable and ensuing community mental health, can be visualized in considering the effect of reduction in the nationwide production of steel on a community with an employment sector heavily concentrated in the steel manufacturing industry. Economic slowdowns in this industrial sector could be predicted to result in mass layoffs and subsequent plant closings. The workers who were primarily trained in steel manufacturing would be faced with significant life stressors, as they would direct efforts toward finding new sources of income to sustain their families. If the plants, the community, or the workers did not have immediate resources for job retraining or if the area did not support other jobs with comparable wages, the commu-

Figure 4-1 ▪ Status of Community Mental Wellness

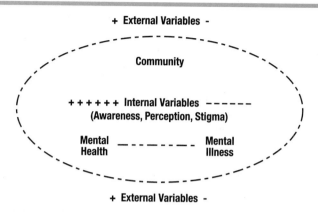

+ External Variables -

Community

+ + + + + + Internal Variables – – – – – –
(Awareness, Perception, Stigma)

Mental _ _ _ _ _ _ _ Mental
Health   Illness

+ External Variables -

Used with permission of Susan Siwinski-Hebel.

nity of workers, families, and the area merchants (who depend upon their daily purchases and trade) would all be faced with significant life stressors. These life stressors would exert pressure upon community members and challenge the maintenance of mental health. Individuals faced with the significant stress of job loss, not to mention the challenge of managing other life stressors such as the care of immediate and/or extended family, fulfilling financial obligations tied to mortgages, maintenance of personal properties, payment of debts, securing resources for secondary education or retirement, or striving to maintain an achieved lifestyle, would encounter the strain upon their ability to manage and cope without a strong, existing support network.

Considering that an individual perceives a state of mental health while contributing to his or her family or society, any prolonged period without work would compromise mental well-being. Under extreme pressures such as these, an individual's usual coping mechanisms frequently become depleted. Compounding risks for reductions in overall mental health, an individual with coping mechanisms that are poorly developed or involve reliance upon external sources of reinforcement is at extreme risk. The possibility for increased risk of isolation, social withdrawal, and increased use of alcohol, drugs, or tobacco is plausible for those with depleted coping reserves. This spiral of loss doesn't just affect adults in the scenario, but impacts children as well. All experience the losses associated with this change and all are subject to reduced mental health.

Needless to say, it is clear to see how a community's overall mental health could be affected by an external variable. Therefore, to garner a clear view of a community's mental wellness status, it is important to involve constituents of the community as well as consider influencing factors in the assessment process. Support for this approach was introduced in the reference to the community-as-partner model from Chapter 1. The model identified components as the constituents, the core of people who create the community, along with eight subsystems that interact through a transactional relationship with the core: the physical environment, community safety, transportation, health and human services, economics, education, politics and government, and recreation (Anderson & McFarlane, 2000). An accurate assessment of mental health requires that needs are examined for all components. External variables (needs) arise from within this multisector region of influence. In other words, the needs emanate from the subsystems. After a thorough assessment has been completed, needs are then incorporated and compared to determine how the findings exert an influence on the community's movement within the mental health and mental illness continuum. Examination of the process justifies further reinforcement for the inclusion of the subsystems in the assessment process, as they provide information about the immediate and potential needs of the community.

Just as there are external variables, internal variables also exist. Exploration of internal variables and the impact exerted upon the mental status of any given community or the individuals therein is required. The degree to which the internal variables of awareness, perception, and stigma exist will have an enhancing or undermining effect on the community's movement toward mental wellness. American communities in general are not the closely intertwined habitats that they were in the 1940s and 1950s. The prevalence of technology and the associated fast-paced lifestyle has influenced how people use their non-working hours in relation to community involvement.

In general, American neighborhoods have become communities of individualism and isolation. Along with this, awareness of other community members' needs has become restricted. In general, people move through each day without a sense of what the major issues are for the community or its members. At the very least, people have chosen to not commit their non-working hours toward community enhancement or participation in local government, community organizations, or affiliations. These choices reduce awareness of potential or real community issues, including mental health issues.

Likewise, perceptions have a tendency to be clouded by increased media reports of violence and dangers lurking within neighborhoods, further limiting a positive impact or drive toward community involvement. Perception of what is known or not known about mental illness can also generate a lack of community member involvement with those individuals who display signs and symptoms of developing or existing mental illness.

Lastly, the prevailing and long-standing stigmas associated with a diagnosis of a mental disorder have kept individuals sequestered from the public at large. Fear and ignorance keep people from accepting members of the community diagnosed with a mental disorder. Literature and movements in treatment have reinforced the benefits to individuals in their rehabilitation and overall health when they are allowed to become integrated members of a community. In recent years there have been strong movements toward group homes for those with **serious mental illnesses (SMI),** chronic mental illness usually found in persons age 18 and older; however, many of these areas of development have been halted because of prevailing stigmatization and resulting community protest.

The interplay of these internal variables has far-reaching effects on community well-being. As a group, the population of the United States has increasingly defined its level of involvement, not only as individuals but also as communities, based on the intrinsic monetary value of the involvement. Failure to initiate involvement in a community's mental health and well-being will lead not only to community health losses, but to the ongoing health loss of each individual even though it may not be readily apparent at this point in time.

Mental health as a community concept was first introduced in the 1960s with the Mental Retardation Facilities and Community Mental Health Centers Construction Act of 1963. Goals of the act were centered on providing comprehensive **mental health services**, interventions for the prevention, diagnosis, and treatment of mental illness. In general, services are geared toward supporting an individual's coping with those issues that threaten maintenance of mental health or improving physical, emotional, and social functioning when mental illness is present. These services are provided to all residents in a specified **catchment area,** a designated service region that encompasses anywhere from 75,000 to 200,000 residents. Corresponding **deinstitutionalization,** the movement of clients diagnosed with mental disorders from state mental hospitals, was the beginning of the shift toward providing community-based mental health services within community settings (families, supervised nursing homes, and apartments). In addition, federal money was made available to states for planning, organizing, and implementing **community mental health centers,** service centers within a specified community created through the joint efforts of federal and state governments to provide services that would intervene with early and intensive treatment for those with mental illness and promote mental health. Treatment teams within centers were formed and comprised of varied health care, psychology, and sociology professionals. A commitment of this proportion further supported our nation's attention and energies toward promoting mental health.

Recent history has witnessed reductions in federal funding and limited state budgets; however, the promotion of mental health for individuals in the community has continued as a valuable goal. The complexity of meeting mental health needs requires and fosters the continued collaboration of treatment teams and disciplines. As part of the charge outlined in the Community Mental Health Center Act of 1963, these centers and affiliated professionals have been mandated to communicate information concerning the representative mental health needs of the designated community or catchment area and to educate others related to those needs. Consultation and education haven't been the centers' only tasks by any means. The extensive roles of providing care to those diagnosed with mental disorders and directing efforts toward ongoing prevention of mental illness has generated disagreement about the purpose of community mental health. Centers, mandated by law, were to provide five essential mental health services: inpatient, emergency, partial hospitalization, outpatient, and consultation and education (Stuart & Laraia, 2001, p. 728). Unfortunately, the planning for deinstitutionalization and the required support services were inadequate and individuals with mental illness often found themselves caught up in a cycle of repeated hospital admissions. In part, the consumer-based mental health promotion and mental illness prevention activities may well have arisen from the massive responsibilities placed upon community mental health centers and the corresponding diminishing availability of financial and personnel resources realized in the past three decades.

During these past decades an expanded concept of meeting community mental health needs has been implemented through the **community support system (CSS)**. CSS is a model for community-based mental health services with multiple components that are primarily developed and implemented by an assigned community mental health center. The services offered include client identification and outreach, mental health treatment, health and dental care, crisis response services, protection and advocacy, rehabilitation, family and community support, peer support, income support, and entitlement and housing (National Institute of Mental Health [NIMH], 1987, as cited in Frisch & Frisch, 1998, p. 705). Legislation has provided more stable funding for the development of CSSs, but difficulties persist in securing consistent financial bases for operation. Increasingly, the growing consumer support and advocacy group movements and involved community organizations find themselves searching for means to meet the needs of their constituents or targeted segments of population. Wherever the level of involvement, there are broad benefits gained through an ability to articulate the needs central to a center's, disciplines', or group's involvement in providing for mental health needs. The exploration of the needs assessment process in the following pages will provide the focus and direction for planning and the foundation for targeted activities.

Additional information that can provide directives and focus for needs assessments can be found through the activities and issues central within the federal government. The congruence between *Healthy People 2010* goals and the activities in motion within the congressional legislative body is evident. Proposed resolutions and bills reinforce that political decision makers are well aware of the crisis communities are facing and the burgeoning mental health needs of the nation. Ever-expanding mental health requirements of the nation and the inconsistencies that abound in an individual's ability to pursue mental as well as physical health services are repetitive themes that resound throughout sessions of Congress. As of this writing, several resolutions and bills have been proposed in both the House of Representatives and the Senate that seek provisions for greater treatment access and equitable insurance coverage to those diagnosed with mental disorders.

House of Representatives Resolution 14 (2001) was presented as a demonstration of awareness and support acknowledging the seriousness of the national problems associated with mental illness and with respect to Congress's intent to establish a Mental Health Advisory Committee. House of Representatives Bill 162 (2001) directs efforts toward amending the Public Health Service Act, Employee Retirement Income Act of 1974, and the Internal Revenue Code of 1986 prohibiting group and individual health plans from imposing treatment limitations or financial requirements on the coverage of mental health benefits and substance abuse and chemical dependency benefits. The bill stipulates that mental health, substance abuse, and chemical dependency benefits can be limited or have certain requirements imposed only when similar restrictions exist within accompanying medical and surgical benefits. House of Representatives Bill 2364 (2001) requires an amendment to title XIX of the Social Security Act that would provide states with an option of covering intensive community mental health treatment under the Medicaid Program. Senate Bill 543 (2001) has been proposed to ensure greater **parity** in the coverage of mental health benefits by prohibiting a group health plan from treating mental health beneficiaries differently than medical and surgical beneficiaries. Parity exists when there is equity between benefits as well as limitations provided under medical, surgical, mental illness, and mental health insurance coverage. Coverage that discriminates based on a diagnosis of a mental disorder or for seeking mental health services would be non-existent if full parity was assured within health insurance. Senate Bill 690 (2001) has proposed to amend title XVIII of the Social Security Act to expand and improve coverage of mental health services under Medicare. Senate Bill 859 (2001) seeks to amend the Public Health Service Act for varied purposes, including the establishment of a mental health community education program that would provide expanded community access to services and education for professionals and community members in rurally designated areas.

These resolutions and bills alert the reader to movements and issues central to changes in access and delivery of mental health services in the nation. It is further recommended that the reader remain aware of these types of government activities to stay abreast of movements and trends in the provision of mental health services, potential projects, or grants that may arise from government decisions. The Library of Congress web site, http://thomas.loc.gov, offers direct links for conducting searches on federal resolutions and bills, with summaries and available status reports for the current session of the United States Congress as well as archival proceedings. The reader should follow the federal issues impacting mental health services and mental illness, such as Medicaid and Supplemental Security Income (SSI), housing, non-discrimination, prison care, health coverage, and mental health block grants. Developments central to mental health and illness can be tracked by reviewing the activities of the presiding legislative committees that have jurisdiction over decisions. These committees include Education and the Workforce, Ways and Means, Judiciary, Commerce, Veteran's Affairs, and Appropriations and Banking (H.R. Res. 14).

Statistics concerning the prevalence of mental illness (discussed in detail in step two of the process model), limitations generated by barriers to accessing mental health care services, and lack of parity in health care coverage are staggering and appalling. In 1996, the Mental Health Parity Act was introduced and the long battle to equate mental health insurance provisions with those provided for medical and surgical coverage began. Initially, parity was only achieved in annual and lifetime limits in care, but the battle lines were drawn with hopes that discrimination would no longer be tolerated. Unfortunately, employers and insurance companies have made the most of the loopholes in the act and manipulated insurance coverage for the treatment of mental illness. Those seeking mental health care coverage have experienced this through increased co-payments and deductible costs, barriers to accessing care, reduced approvals for hospital admissions and outpatient treatment days, and refusals for coverage.

"The United States General Accounting Office issued a report in May, 2000, that verified that despite passage of the 1996 mental health parity law, 14 percent of employers failed to comply with even the limited protections required by law. Of the 86 percent that did comply, most (87%) continued to limit their mental health benefits" (S. 543, p. S235). Another legislative attempt to correct this disparity resides in the Mental Health Equitable Treatment Act of 2001. The act would provide full parity for all mental disorders listed in the *Diagnostic and Statistical Manual of Mental Disorders 4th edition* (DSM IV), the primary standard by which mental disorders are diagnosed in the United States. Mental illnesses having similar characteristics are grouped into 16 major diagnostic classes. Each disorder within a class is organized according to the specific signs, symptoms, and patterns of criteria that are needed to conduct a diagnostic evaluation. In addition to the broad coverage provisions for mental disorders, the Mental Health Equitable Treatment Act of 2001 prohibits group health plans from forcing treatment limitations that are different from other medical and surgical benefits. Despite the act, a potential deficit may yet arise. Mandated mental health benefits would not be secured within all beneficiaries' health insurance packages; parity would only be realized through those group plans that already offered mental health coverage (S. 543, p. S236).

STEPS OF THE MENTAL HEALTH AND WELLNESS ASSESSMENT

Four goals of *Healthy People 2010* addressing the assessment and functioning of mental health and well-being are presented and discussed in this chapter. These goals were selected for an overall interrelationship and impact upon mental health. Goal 18, addressing the improvement of mental health and associated services, has a direct relationship to mental well-being. Subsequently, goal 22, addressing physical activity, is included in this section. The degree that a community demonstrates engagement in physical activity can be correlated with the community's adaptation potential in the presence of stressors. These potential adaptive coping mechanisms can be interpreted as enhancements to the maintenance or restoration of mental health within the overall community. The other two goals, 26 and 27, relate to bringing about reductions in the use of addictive substances. These substances are used by community members as maladaptive coping mechanisms in the presence of stressors and are associated with consequences of illness and mortality. Furthermore, the relationships between goals are reinforced through the parallel presentation of contributing ancillary goals and objectives (see Table 4-1).

TABLE 4-1 Healthy People 2010 Goal Related to Mental Health and Wellness

GOAL #	GENERAL TOPIC	HEALTHY PEOPLE 2010 GOAL	RELATED HEALTHY PEOPLE 2010 GOALS & OBJECTIVES
18	Mental health	Improve mental health and access to appropriate, quality mental health services.	*Substance Abuse* 26–7. Alcohol and drug-related violence 26–8. Lost productivity 26–9. Substance-free youth 26–10. Adolescent and adult use of illicit substances 26–11. Binge drinking 26–12. Average annual alcohol consumption 26–13. Low-risk drinking among adults 26–14. Steroid use among adolescents 26–15. Inhalant use among adolescents 26–16. Peer disapproval of substance abuse 26–17. Perception of risk associated with substance abuse 26–18. Treatment gap for illicit drugs 26–22. Hospital emergency department referrals 26–23. Community partnerships and coalitions
22	Physical activity	Improve health, fitness, and quality of life through daily physical activity.	*Mental Health and Mental Disorders* 18–5. Eating disorder relapse 18–7. Treatment for children with mental health problems 18–9. Treatment for adults with mental disorders *Substance Abuse* 26–9. Substance-free youth 26–14. Steroid use among adolescents

| 26 | Substance abuse | Reduce substance abuse to protect the health, safety, and quality of life for all, especially children. | 26-17. Perception of risk associated with substance abuse
26-23. Community partnerships and coalitions
Tobacco Use
27-1. Adult tobacco use
27-2. Adolescent tobacco use
27-3. Initiation of tobacco use
27-4. Age at first tobacco use
27-5. Smoking cessation by adults
27-7. Smoking cessation by adolescents
Mental Health and Mental Disorders
18-6. Primary care screening and assessment
18-10. Treatment for co-occurring disorders
18-13. Treatment for adults with mental disorders
Tobacco Use
27-1. Adult tobacco use
27-2. Adolescent tobacco use
27-3. Initiation of tobacco use
27-4. Age at first tobacco use
27-5. Smoking cessation by adults
27-6. Smoking cessation during pregnancy
27-7. Smoking cessation by adolescents
27-8. Insurance coverage of cessation treatment
27-9. Exposure to tobacco smoke at home among children
27-10. Exposure to environmental tobacco smoke
27-11. Smoke-free and tobacco-free schools
27-12. Worksite smoking policies |

continues

TABLE 4-1 Healthy People 2010 Goal Related to Mental Health and Wellness *continued*

GOAL #	GENERAL TOPIC	HEALTHY PEOPLE 2010 GOAL	RELATED HEALTHY PEOPLE 2010 GOALS & OBJECTIVES
			27–13. Smoke-free indoor air laws
			27–14. Enforcement of illegal tobacco sales to minors laws
			27–15. Retail license suspension for sales to minors
			27–16. Tobacco advertising and promotion targeting adolescents and young adults
			27–17. Adolescent disapproval of smoking
			27–18. Tobacco control programs
			27–19. Preemptive tobacco control laws
			27–20. Tobacco product regulation
			27–21. Tobacco tax
27	Tobacco use	Reduce illness, disability, and death related to tobacco use and exposure to secondhand smoke.	*Substance Abuse*
			26–9. Substance-free youth
			26–16. Peer disapproval of substance abuse
			26–17. Perception of risk associated with substance abuse

Throughout section three on information gathering, each goal's importance is reinforced and the relationship to mental health and wellness is explored. Information is also cited as to where resources on the associated issues are located.

Step One: Definition and Description of the Needs Assessment Problem

In the past, mental health needs assessments have been broad and unyielding. The literature suggests that there has been a deficit in pinpointing specific mental health needs of a targeted group. In general, there has been a tendency on the part of the assessing body to develop their own testing instruments rather than using those already established as scientifically credible and valid. Furthermore, those pursuing needs assessments have frequently been at a disadvantage, as there has been a lack of specific standards to apply and an absence of identified goals to pursue. Some authors (Royse & Drude, 1982) delivered a call for greater uniformity in needs assessment approaches, a distinct focus for needs assessments, and macro-level collaboration among related mental health agencies.

While federal health planning and accountability efforts have led to regional planning (i.e., health systems agencies) and regional service reviews (i.e., professional standards review organizations), there has not been comparable development for mental health. Federal and state legislation for mental health should more explicitly promote comprehensive and integrative approaches to the identification of mental health service needs at the regional level or multiple mental health service areas. Although federal and state health planning agencies have technically been responsible for physical and mental health needs assessment, mental health has tended to get much less emphasis than physical health (Royse & Drude, 1995, p. 102).

Combining the Ontario Needs Impact Based Model with the goals, objectives, and benchmarks of *Healthy People 2010,* and eliciting the collaboration of community leaders, agency representatives, or interested members of the community is one way to rectify the disparity in conducting assessments and render findings that can be generalized and integrated. Considering the needs of a targeted group, return to the three areas that constitute representative needs identified in the Ontario model, expressed, felt, and normative. Having representation from a broad cross-section would not only assist in communication of these needs, but would go a long way toward creating overall community investment. Furthermore, the incorporation of the related *Healthy People 2010* goals within mental health needs assessment creates focus and structure.

Aside from the recommended point of focus and a consistent approach among all those involved in conducting a needs assessment, there is additional evidence that supports the fostering of a mutual working relationship among agencies that track similar data or provide related services. Frequently, the process of establishing interagency collaborative relationships proves to be difficult because of agency policies, procedures, and mandates; however, it is an alliance with other groups having similar interests that provides multiple gains. **Key stakeholders,** individuals responsible for the development and administration of mental health services provided to children, adults, and families within specified regions and populations, have a vested interest in collaborating, especially poignant considering the reality of limited health care funding, budgets, and resources. After all, the overarching benefit of collaboration will be experienced by all participants involved in a joint effort, as individuals who develop multidimensional mental health needs access services from a multitude of providers throughout their lifetime. A model for this kind of collaboration was developed and implemented by a partnership group in DuPage County in Illinois. A coalition convened to conduct a community-specific needs assessment to assist in determining interventions for children and youth with emotional or behavioral disorders and their families.

The partnership was established and joint information gathering processes were developed, putting in place a three-tier process (archival review of case records for demographics, risk factor analysis, and criterion-referenced searches of relevant agency selected case studies) to ensure all parties were afforded inclusion and that the data was cross-sectional and longitudinal across all agencies. In addition, surveys of service providers, parents, and agency key stakeholders were conducted. Lastly, the group cooperatively engaged in the analysis and synthesis of the data as well as the generation of an action plan. Many benefits from this type of approach were realized. The partnership afforded members the ability to submit an alternative funding plan to their state agencies, began a new vision for the flexible use of service funds, allowed direct service staff to experience the benefits of working in interagency teams, promoted coordination of services across agencies, generated case management plans that focused on the return of children who were in out-of-state placement, engaged private providers in a community treatment approach, set the stage for submission of a grant proposal for the establishment of an early intervention program, demonstrated need necessary for securing funding for volunteers and respite services, and created an integrated system of services to children and families that spanned previously impervious agency barriers (Epstein, Quinn, Cumblad, & Holderness, 1996; Quinn, Epstein, Cumblad,

& Holderness, 1996). In applying this model along with the process of the Ontario Needs Impact Based Model and *Healthy People 2010,* a strong foundation to pursue funding for targeted interventions is built.

A personal account of the identification of a specific community mental health problem, outlined as the initial step of the Ontario Needs Impact Based Model, is offered for direct application. I was a member of the group referenced in the preface to this book; thus, my experience with the process outlined in the model is explored. An active, dynamic community advocate approached a nursing faculty seeking support in the development of a proposal that would meet the needs of people with early memory loss. The individual was passionate about the perceived need and had already been searching for support and collaboration from various community health providers. In this case it was a community member who was instrumental in identifying the problem. Specifically, it was perceived that there was a population of individuals within the community who were experiencing or diagnosed with early onset memory loss that would benefit from peer support or counseling services. The problem statement can be defined as "What segment of the population would benefit from a support group for people with early onset memory loss?" Contributing members of the assessment group engaged in ongoing exploration and dialogue with the community advocate and a specific, detailed purpose and proposal was created. The proposal sought to develop a support group for people experiencing early memory loss and suggested three types of services: (1) a peer support group, facilitated by a dementia educator or health care provider, which could enhance quality of life by supporting and prolonging social and cognitive functioning; (2) a directory of trained faculty, staff, student, and community volunteers that could provide dementia education and support services through area disability, aging, and rehabilitation agencies; and (3) consultants identified through the project that could work with area agencies or community leaders to develop innovative models of care that would support the dignity and maximize the independence and functioning of people with dementia. In this scenario, the ongoing process of assessment became important in supporting the perceptions driving the proposal and instrumental in demonstrating sustainability of a designated mental health service.

Step Two: Determining What Information Is Required

The process of initiating the assessment of a community's mental health and well-being begins by focusing on original priorities that were targeted within *Healthy People 2000.* Lead agencies, the Substance Abuse and Mental Health Services Administration (SAMHSA) and National

Institute of Mental Health (NIMH), were commissioned with the task of setting the priorities. The following objectives were identified:

- Reduce the number of suicides.
- Reduce the incidence of injurious suicide attempts among adolescents.
- Reduce the prevalence of mental disorders among children and adolescents.
- Reduce the prevalence of mental disorders among adults living in the community.
- Reduce adverse effects from stress.
- Increase use of community support programs by people with severe, persistent mental disorders.
- Increase use of treatment by people with major depressive disorders.
- Increase number of people who seek help for personal and emotional problems.
- Reduce uncontrolled stress.
- Increase appropriate prevention strategies for suicide by jail inmates.
- Increase worksite stress prevention programs.
- Establish mutual help clearinghouses.
- Increase routine reviews of cognitive, emotional, and behavioral functioning by primary care providers for adults.
- Increase routine reviews of cognitive, emotional, and behavioral functioning by primary care providers for children.
- Reduce the prevalence of depressive disorders among adults.

(U.S. Department of Health and Human Services, 1995).

Additional priorities addressing physical activity and fitness and tobacco and substance abuse (alcohol and other drugs) were included, just as they are in the 2010 initiative. In reviewing Table 4-1, there is evidence of transference from the *Healthy People 2000* mental health and mental disorders priorities and objectives to the continuing *Healthy People 2010* goals and objectives. In July 1999, a final review of the overall progress in achieving the objectives for mental health and mental disorders was conducted. Discussions revealed that the issues of **resilience,** a personal trait or characteristic that contributes to an individual's ability to develop coping resources, adapt, and become competent in managing the stressors of life, access and availability of quality care in evolving delivery models, and the impact of mental disorders upon the Global Burden of Disease were prevailing and paramount throughout all the collected statistics (U.S. Department of Health and Human Services, 1999).

In support of data and statistics that correlate with the direction laid out by *Healthy People 2010,* a general review of the epidemiology relating to mental disorders that has been collected and presented in two notable studies is shared: the Epidemiologic Catchment Area (ECA) study and the National Comorbidity Survey (NCS). They were both conducted during the early 1990s, the ECA in 1991 and the NCS in 1994, with relatively large samples, but different populations. The findings revealed "one third to one half of all adults in the United States will have a mental disorder in their lifetime" (Fortinash & Holoday-Worret, 2000, p. 9).

In the ECA survey, researchers from NIMH interviewed almost 20,000 adults in multiple sites to establish the one-year and lifetime prevalence of 30 mental disorders. Researchers from the NCS interviewed 8,098 adults regarding 17 of the most commonly occurring disorders. The ECA and NCS concluded that mental disorders affected approximately 20 percent to 30 percent of adults in the United States during the year preceding the interviews and 32 percent to 50 percent throughout their lives (Robins & Regier, 1991; Kessler et al, 1994; and Maxman & Ward, 1995, as cited in Fortinash, & Holoday-Worret, 2000, p. 9).

In reviewing readily available online statistics published through NIMH, the following gender differences were noted:

◆ Nearly twice as many women (12.0 percent) as men (6.6 percent) are affected by a depressive disorder each year.

◆ The highest suicide rates in the United States are found in white men over age 85.

◆ Four times more men than women commit suicide; however, women attempt suicide two to three times as often as men.

◆ Women are more likely than men to have an anxiety disorder.

◆ Approximately two times more women than men suffer from panic disorder, post-traumatic stress disorder, generalized anxiety disorder, agoraphobia, and specific phobias, although about equal numbers of women and men have obsessive-compulsive disorder and social phobia.

◆ Females are much more likely than males to develop an eating disorder.

◆ Only an estimated 5 to 15 percent of people with anorexia or bulimia and a small percent of those with binge-eating disorder are male.

♦ About two to three times more boys than girls are affected with attention deficit hyperactivity disorder (ADHD).

♦ Autism is about four times more common in boys than girls; Girls with the disorder, however, tend to have more severe symptoms and greater cognitive impairment (NIMH, 2001).

Of all the diagnosable mental disorders, depression is the leading cause of disability. Three other disorders, bipolar disorder, schizophrenia, and obsessive-compulsive disorder, are within the top 10 causes of disability. NIMH identifies depression as a critical public health problem. More than 18 million people in the United States will suffer from a depressive illness in the current year, and many will experience the debilitation of the illness and consequences that affect their ability to work and contribute to the care of their families (NIMH, 2001). The cost of mental illness to the United States is staggering and frequently cited in the billions of dollars while the total impact of burden and suffering cannot be calculated into statements of financial loss.

The direct costs of mental health services in the United States in 1996 totaled $69.0 billion. This figure represents 7.3 percent of total health spending. An additional $17.7 billion was spent on Alzheimer's disease and $12.6 billion on substance abuse treatment. Direct costs correspond to spending for treatment and rehabilitation nationwide. Indirect costs can be defined in different ways . . . lost productivity at the workplace, school, and home due to premature death or disability. The indirect costs of mental illness were estimated in 1990 at $78.6 billion. More than 80 percent of these costs stemmed from disability rather than death because mortality from mental disorders is relatively low (Rice & Miller, 1996, as cited in U.S. Department of Health and Human Services, 1999).

Despite the impact upon adults in the United States, children are experiencing exceptional barriers arising from the effects of mental disorders. While suicide is an objective focused on for the mental health of adolescents in *Healthy People 2010,* recent legislation and news reports have been focused on children with emotional and behavioral disorders (EBD) that are a precursor of SMI. The fragmentation of service, issues of abandonment, and community rejection that these children and their families are experiencing are devastating. "The 1998 *Surgeon General's Report on Mental Health* estimates that between five and nine percent of those under age eighteen have mental disorders so severe that they face overwhelming difficulties in the efforts to function well with their families, friends, and teachers" (Mental Health Equitable, 2001, p. S235). Further support for this skyrocketing need is documented as more and more children and adolescents are identified as a population at risk within our school systems and are subsequently diagnosed with EBD. There are grave concerns that social agencies, given their current policies, procedures, and practices, are not in a position to advocate for children with serious EBD to be retained not only in their communities, but also within their families. It is difficult to ascertain how many parents nationwide have had to give up custody to get services to provide everyday care to their children. "Critics contend that government programs and private insurers discriminate when they set tight payment limits for children with severe mental disabilities . . . limits they don't set for children with long-term physical illnesses. There is entitlement for nursing home or institutional placement, but not to live within the community . . . it becomes an issue of cost, profits, and jobs" (Silberner, 2001).

A comprehensive assessment of mental health and well-being also requires recognition of the targeted population's cultural identity. It is noted that within a group the cultural identity of its individual members "may also involve language, country of origin, acculturation (social distance separating members of an ethnic or racial group from the larger society), gender, age, class, religious/spiritual beliefs, sexual orientation, and physical disabilities" (Lu et al., 1995, as cited in U.S. Department of Health and Human Services, 1999, p. 81). In general, reports have shown that the United States is not proficient in meeting the mental health needs of diverse cultures. In assessing the needs of the unique cultures within a community, one must recognize that along with a cultural identity comes "distinct patterns of beliefs and practices that have implications for the willingness to seek, and the ability to respond to mental health services. These include coping styles and ties to family and community" (U.S. Department of Health and Human Services, 1999, p. 82). Therefore, including recommendations and feedback from recognized leaders or members who are representative of cultural segments is mandatory in achieving a detailed and culturally sensitive assessment.

Associated with the running example presented throughout this chapter, the following information elucidates step one's problem statement, providing further direct guidance in the assessment process. Upon reviewing the *Healthy People 2010* focus areas, a linkage was made with the problem statement and goal 18: "Improve mental health and ensure access to appropriate, quality mental health services" (U.S. Department of Health and Human Services, 2000, p. 18–3); next, with a centering objective, 18–6: "Increase the number of persons seen in primary health care who receive mental health screening and assessment" (U.S. Department of Health and Human Services, 2000, p. 18–16). This objective is developmental, subsequently, there is no target data to benchmark the need against for evaluation. Furthermore, a foundation for understanding the development and incidence of early memory loss is needed before further assessment proceeds.

Onset of early memory loss, associated with the development of dementia, can be related to a variety of causes. Dementia refers to "the general syndrome of acquired and intellectual impairment caused by dysfunction. The syndrome of dementia involves persistent impairment of two or more of the following domains of psychological functioning: memory, language, visuospatial skills, judgment or abstract thinking, and emotion or personality" (Storandt & Vandenbos, 1995, p. 85). Because of the difficulties practitioners have had in the process of establishing a definitive diagnosis in the early stages (usually diagnosed as depression in the early stages), the actual prevalence of the syndrome is unknown. "Average prevalence estimates across studies suggest that approximately 6% of persons over the age of 65 years have severe dementia, with an additional 10–15% having mild-to-moderate dementias" (Cummings & Benson, 1992 as cited in Storandt & Vandenbos, 1995, p. 85).

In addition to multiple causes, age and corresponding disease process can be the impetus for the syndrome. Alzheimer's disease (DAT) is the stimulus for up to "75% of all dementia cases in people over the age of 60. Other causes (that can occur at any age) include multiple strokes or vascular dementia (VaD), Huntington's disease, Parkinson's disease, Pick's disease, multiple sclerosis, and many others. The so-called 'reversible' causes of dementia include vitamin B12 deficiency, hypothyroidism, neurosyphillis, and possibly hyperparathyroidism" (*Alzheimer's frequently discussed topics,* 1995). Little research has been done on the prevalence of early onset dementia in those under age 65. A recent study conducted over a two-and-a-half-year period in two London boroughs used a comprehensive methodology in an attempt to identify cases of dementia that began before age 65 and the related causes. The study identified 185 cases of young onset dementia, giving a prevalence of 67.2 cases per 100,000 at risk in the 30–64 age group. Furthermore the researchers concluded that the younger group of patients diagnosed with dementia appeared to be less likely to use community resources and depended upon more costly institutional care. Over the period of this study, an amplified concern about and services for younger people developed (Dementia Research Group, 1998).

Several secondary questions are posed considering the above information and providing direction for the information gathering process: What is the incidence of those people diagnosed with early memory loss in the region? What is the general population's awareness of the identification of signs and symptoms associated with early memory loss? What percentage of primary care health professionals screen for the presence of early memory loss?

Step Three: Information Gathering

Information to substantiate mental health needs can be gathered through a variety of means and resources. As mentioned in other chapters, online computer searching for supporting data is a plentiful and efficient retrieval method. Many of the electronic resources used in the development of this chapter and recommended to the reader have built-in search features on the web site homepage. State and federal government agencies have massive databases that allow searches according to dates, issues, and key words. In addition, data from key informants representing service agencies, community service organizations, and social institutions provides valuable information that builds a well-rounded assessment. The remainder of this section explores the nuances of four goals from *Healthy People 2010* that correspond to mental health and wellness and identifies suggested resources for data gathering.

Goal Eighteen: Mental Health

Goal 18 is to "Improve mental health and access to appropriate, quality mental health services" (U.S. Department of Health and Human Services, 2000, p. 18–3). There are 14 objectives associated with this goal. The objectives relate to the incidence of suicide within the population as a whole and among adolescents in particular. The prevalence of homelessness among those diagnosed with SMI and the employment rates among those with SMI are included. Identification of interventions to reduce relapse rates for eating disorder relapses are targeted. Expansion of treatment services are also a priority through increases made in primary screening and assessment for the general public and within juvenile justice facilities, services provided to children with mental health problems, services provided to adults with mental disorders and co-occurring disorders, and adult jail diversion programs. Lastly, establishment and improvements in state tracking systems of consumer satisfaction, cultural competency, and plans addressing elderly persons are sought (U.S. Department of Health and Human Services, 2000). Box 4-1 lists available resources pertaining to goal 18 that were current as of this writing

Goal Twenty-Two: Physical Activity

Goal 22 seeks to "Improve health, fitness, and quality of life through daily physical activity" (U.S. Department of Health and Human Services, 2000, p. 22–3). There are 15 objectives associated with this goal. The objectives relating to physical activity in adults and children acknowledge the

---

Box 4-1 ■ Information Resources for Mental Health

*National Alliance for the Mentally Ill (NAMI)—
http://www.nami.org/level.html*

*National Mental Health Association (NMHA)—
http://www.nmha.org/*

*Mental health:A report of the Surgeon General—http://www.sur-
geongeneral.gov/library/mentalhealth/home.html*

Bazelon Center for Mental Health Law—http://www.bazelon.org/

*National Association of State Mental Health Planning Directors
(NASMHPD)—http://www.nasmhpd.org*

---

known historical benefits to physical health, but the far-reaching benefits
of overall fitness and enhanced quality of life are now also targeted for improvement. The focus is not only on the preventative benefits, but also on
the protective benefits. Related to mental well-being, a Surgeon General's
report from 1996 cited evidence supporting the enhancement effects
upon mental health. "Aerobic physical activities, such as brisk walking and
running, were found to improve mental health for people who report
symptoms of anxiety and depression and for those who are diagnosed
with some forms of depression" (U.S. Department of Health and Human
Services, 1999, p. 232). The objectives within this goal specifically seek to
improve the mental health of adults engaging in leisure-time, moderate,
and vigorous physical activities. Enhancements to overall muscular
strength, muscular endurance, and flexibility are also sought. Improvement can be gained by addressing the physical activity among children
and adolescents through increased moderate and vigorous activities and
reductions in television viewing. Primary schools are included in these objectives by efforts undertaken to expand requirements for physical education, offering regular outlets for activity, and incorporating more
physical activity, in physical education classes (U.S. Department of Health
and Human Services, 2000, p. 22–7). Lastly, the objectives focus on access
to school facilities, workplace promotion of physical activity and expanded efforts to promote walking and bicycling as feasible modes of
transportation (U.S. Department of Health and Human Services, 2000).
There are resources that offer information in this area available at federal,
state, and local levels of the government, such as the Centers for Disease

Control and Prevention (CDC) and the National Center for Healthcare Statistics (NCHS). Public and private school system administrators are also a source of data. Lastly, local and state park departments and chambers of commerce have leisure and recreational data and a *Nationwide Personal Transportation Survey* offers data that supports investigation in this area.

Goal Twenty-Six: Substance Abuse

Goal 26 seeks to "Reduce substance abuse to protect the health, safety, and quality of life for all, especially children" (U.S. Department of Health and Human Services, 2000, p. 26–3). There are 21 objectives related to this goal. The problems associated with substance abuse are among the most severe in our communities. The far-reaching social implications and adverse health effects are of great concern. Among populations being targeted, adolescents and young adults remain at high risk. While overall drug use has declined, "use among adolescents aged twelve to seventeen years doubled between 1992 and 1997, from 5.3 percent to 11.4 percent" (U.S. Department of Health and Human Services, 2000, p. 26–5). As far as identifying data that demonstrates a relationship between substance use and mental health, a direct correlation with diminished health status has been shown. "Approximately 15 percent of all adults who have a mental disorder in one year also experience a co-occurring substance (alcohol or other drug) use disorder, which complicates treatment" (U.S. Department of Health and Human Services, 1999, p. 15). In general, these objectives seek to reduce adverse consequences of substance use and abuse through reductions in accidents and deaths related to motor vehicle crashes, cirrhosis (a severe disease of the liver), drug-induced incidents, drug- and alcohol-related hospital emergency visits, adolescents taking transportation with intoxicated drivers, alcohol and drug-related violence, and lost productivity. Reduction of substance use and abuse is sought by increasing the numbers of substance-free youth, diminishing adult and adolescent use of illicit substances, binge drinking, steroid and inhalant use, as well as decreasing low-risk drinking among adults. Finally, risk of substance use and abuse can be countered through peer intervention and reinforcement of negative perceptions associated with use. Treatment for substance abuse should be expanded by lessening the gaps in services targeting use of illicit drugs, services provided in correctional facilities, services for those who inject drugs, and problem alcohol use (U.S. Department of Health and Human Services, 2000). Resources are available through the Drug Prevention Resource Center Indiana University Statistics web site on alcohol, tobacco, and other drug use and prevention planning demographics. Links to full-text reports and tables can be accessed through http://www.drugs.indiana.edu/drug_stats/indiana.html. Additional resources on federal and state vital statistics are available through CDC, NCHS, and the Youth Risk Behavior Surveillance System as well as the Substance Abuse and Mental Health Services Administration (SAMHSA).

Goal Twenty-Seven: Tobacco Use

Goal 27 is to "Reduce illness, disability, and death related to tobacco use and exposure to secondhand smoke" (U.S. Department of Health and Human Services, 2000, p. 27–9). There are 21 objectives targeting tobacco use in adult and adolescent population groups, smoking cessation among adults, adolescents, and during pregnancy along with insurance coverage for treatment, exposure to secondhand smoke in residences with children, tobacco and smoke-free schools, and general environmental exposure while reinforcing worksite smoking policies and supporting smoke-free indoor air legislation. Social and environmental changes include adherence to legislation that bans illegal tobacco sales to minors and suspension of retail licenses for those sales. A reduction in advertising and promotion targeting adolescents and tobacco control programs, anticipatory laws, product regulation, and taxes are also integrated within these objectives (U.S. Department of Health and Human Services, 2000). Resources for this information can be found through the CDC, NCHS, the Youth Risk Behavior Surveillance System, and SAMHSA.

Again, tying into the running chapter example, resources for additional data to substantiate comparative and expressed mental health needs, using *Healthy People* goal 18, objective 6, could be obtained from online data retrieval (see Table 4-2), surveys and interviews with providers of primary health care services as well as psychiatric and mental health service providers, existing support groups for caregivers of those individuals diagnosed with DAT, corporate employee assistance programs, community mental health service organizations, hospitals, assisted and skilled living facilities and facilities that offer respite services.

Step Four: Analysis of the Information

The preceding steps of the assessment process applied within this chapter have provided the reader with ample data for consideration and application to any unique problem involving community mental health and well-being. Referencing the targets set within each *Healthy People*

TABLE 4-2 Data Resources for Alzheimer's Disease and Dementia

WEBSIDE	LINK
ADEAR-Alzheimer's Disease Education and Referral Center	http://www.alzheimers.org/
Alzheimer's Disease Menu	http://dem0nmac.mgh.harvard.edu/neurowebforum/ AlzheimersDiseaseMenu.html
Alzheimer Page	http://www.biostat.wustl.edu/alzheimer/
Alzheimer Web Home Page	http://home.mira.net/~dhs/ad.html
CANDID-Counseling and Diagnosis in Dementia	http://dementia.ion.ucl.ac.uk/
Indiana Alzheimer Disease Center National Cell Repository	http://www.iupui.edu/~medgen/research/alz/ alzheimer.html
Medical and Molecular Genetics Home Page	http://www.iupui.edu/~medgen/home2.html

2010 objective and engaging in comparisons to benchmarked data refutes or corroborates the identified problem. Two examples, one specific and the other broad, are presented below.

In conducting an analysis of goal 18, objective 6, through retrieval of data connected to the prevailing problem statement identified as the running example throughout this chapter, there is evidence reinforcing the need for increased efforts to screen for mental health needs. Screening can contribute to the subsequent detection of deficits indicating signs and symptoms of early memory loss. This point is crucial not only in the timely management of early memory loss, but in providing valuable information that helps to refine data collection around the developed problem statement.

The 1998 U.S. Surgeon General's report on mental health stated that "Alzheimer's disease and other dementias are currently underrecognized, especially in primary care settings, where most older patients seek care. The reasons for primary care provider difficulty with diagnosis are speculated to include lack of knowledge or skills, misdiagnosis of depression as dementia, lack of time and lack of adequate referrals to specialty mental health care" (U.S. Department of Human Services, 1999, p. 358). This information further guides the assessment team in developing secondary surveys and interviews that are sensitive to the above components. In addition, this information presents further support for the development of an early memory loss support group that can be a point of referral for practitioners, identifying those individuals with the mild symptoms of dementia who lack resources to aid them in gaining knowledge, understanding, and reinforcement of coping in managing daily life changes.

Data was also gathered that gave insight into a specific cultural component and issues affecting accessibility. Considering the cultural component of this specific assessment, information was presented at the 10th National Alzheimer's Disease Education Conference in Chicago, Illinois, pertinent to the African American culture within the targeted Midwestern region. Results of two African American focus group sessions on Alzheimer caregivers' opinions of the health care system revealed that there "was a belief that physicians were not aware of local services that could help families" (*Alzheimer's Disease: African-Americans at Risk,* July 20, 2001, p. 5). Ongoing data collection revealed that there were no groups that specifically targeted early onset memory loss within the region. Similarly, as referenced in data cited from a study that was presented earlier in this chapter, most of the focus is currently centered on assisted living facilities and premature nursing home placement. Effective intervention to delay onset of early memory loss and enhance coping would be significantly less expensive to taxpayers than placement in expensive assisted or skilled living facilities. The only existing support groups, targeting dementia (or more commonly DAT), provide much needed services across a broad range of issues for the caregivers of those diagnosed family members, significant others, or friends. Furthermore, it appears that support groups for people with early memory loss are only located within the major neighboring, metropolitan areas such as Chicago, Illinois, and Indianapolis, Indiana, further limiting regional access by travel time and traffic congestion.

Table 4-3 conveys the findings of an assessment targeting the current state of mental health in a tricounty Midwestern region of the United States. Status and progress toward *Healthy People 2010* goal 18 is highlighted. The table demonstrates improvements in targets, quality, and overall access to services. The key indicator findings are depicted within seven objectives, related comparative data, indication of identified need, and recommendations. The data concerning this one goal indicates that all relevant objectives have not been met, either because a need was clearly indicated or because the indicated data was not readily available

TABLE 4-3 Example: Needs Assessment: Mental Health and Wellness

Goal Eighteen: Improve Mental Health and Access to Appropriate, Quality Mental Health Services.

HP 2010 OBJECTIVES	TARGET	DATA ASSESSED	NEED	RECOMMENDATIONS
1. Reduce the suicide rate.	To 5% per population of 100,000.	In 1997 the age-adjusted death rates from suicide in the following midwestern counties were: Lake—8.23; LaPorte—16.16; and Porter—9.04 (Indiana Hospital Consumer Guide, 1996–1997). For females in Indiana in 1998, suicide was . . . the third leading cause of death for ages 15–24, the fifth leading cause of death for ages 25–34; the fourth leading cause of death for ages 35–44; the eighth leading cause of death for ages 45–54 (National Center for Injury Prevention and Control, 2000).	X	1a. Develop a regional health and wellness center, affiliated with area hospitals, to meet primary mental health needs of the underserved with a specific focus on suicide prevention & wellness counseling services. 1b. Institute immediate efforts to target the needs of females, 15–24 yrs.old, (ages of those present within the physical setting proposed for the regional health and wellness center) through education and wellness counseling. 1c. Conduct additional research of needs of the male gender.
2. Reduce the rate of suicide attempts by adolescents.	To 12-month average of 1%.	Data from the National Youth Risk Behavior Survey for the years 1991–1999 demonstrate the following national trends: rate of students who ever seriously considered suicide has decreased from a high of 29.0% in 1991 to 19.3% in 1999;	X	2a. Form a coalition with area schools to support efforts to increase suicide prevention among female age groups identified at risk. 2b. See 1b. & 1c. 2c. Work with area mental health providers & agencies to disseminate

continues

TABLE 4-3 Example: Needs Assessment: Mental Health and Wellness *continued*

HP 2010 OBJECTIVES	TARGET	DATA ASSESSED	NEED	RECOMMENDATIONS
		rate of attempted suicide has increased slightly from 7.3% in 1992 to 8.3% in 1999 (Youth Risk Behavior Survey, 1999). For females in Indiana in 1998, suicide was the sixth leading cause of death for ages 10–14; the third leading cause of death for ages 15–24 . . . (National Center for Injury Prevention and Control, 2000).		information on the risk factors associated with increased suicide attempts.
3. Reduce the proportion of homeless adults who have SMI.	To 19%	No data available	?	3a. Engage in a longitudinal study with agency key stakeholders and mental health service providers to identify the number of homeless adults with SMI in catchment areas and changes in their state of mental wellbeing, level of functioning and integration into the surrounding communities. 3b. The Indiana Family and Social Services Administration (IFSSA)—Indiana Division of Mental Health has instituted the Olmstead Data Collec-

Objective	Target	Data		Strategies
4. Increase the proportion of persons with (SMI) who are employed.	To 51%	In 1999, 47% of adults receiving treatment from Southlake Center for Mental Health in Lake County worked outside of the home (Southlake Center for Mental Health Annual Report, 1999).	X	tion Tool and further discussion with agency representatives may demonstrate that data is available (IFSSA, 2001). 4a. Identify rates of employment for those persons diagnosed with SMI and serviced within all corresponding regional mental health agency catchment areas. 4b. See 3b.
5. Increase the proportion of adults with mental disorders who receive treatment.	Serious mental illness to 55% 18–54 yrs. Recognized depression to 50% ≥ 18 yrs. Diagnosis of schizophrenia to 75% ≥ 18 yrs. Diagnosis of generalized anxiety disorder to 50% ≥ 18 yrs.	In Lake county in 1996, 9.4% of adults used or tried to access local mental health services or programs, compared to 9.8% nationally (Lake County Health Care Priorities, 1996). In 1995, 33.2% of Gary adults had experienced 2 or more years of depression at some time in their life; which increases to over 46% among adults living below the national poverty level. 9.4% have sought professional help for a mental or emotional problem, compared to 12.9% of Merrillville adults, 9.4% of Lake County adults and 9.9% of	X	5a. Establish a coalition with health care providers; points of ambulatory care services and community outreach services to increase early identification and education, which will support symptom recognition, diagnosis and treatment. 5b. Determine the progress on a statewide database that will collect disease specific data to determine how these disorders will be tracked and how county representation will be differentiated (IDEM and Public Health Subcommittee of the Environmental Quality Service Council, 1999).

continues

TABLE 4-3 Example: Needs Assessment: Mental Health and Wellness *continued*

HP 2010 OBJECTIVES	TARGET	DATA ASSESSED	NEED	RECOMMENDATIONS
		U.S. adults (PRC Community Health Assessment, 1996). In Lake county in 1996, 22.8% of adults faced or had faced bouts with prolonged depression compared to 22.1% nationally. The rate was 44.4% for Lake county adults living below the poverty level (Lake County Health Care Priorities, 1996). In Lake county, 1997 population estimates show that 22,490 people suffer from major depression (Health Resources, 2000). The Surgeon General estimates that 20% of U.S. population is affected by mental disorders during any one year, and 7.1% have a mood disorder; about 1.5% has a diagnosis of schizophrenia or other psychosis; and 16.4% suffer from an anxiety disorder (Mental health: A report of the Surgeon General, 1999).		

6. Increase the number of States and the District of Columbia that track consumers' satisfaction with the mental health services they receive.	50 States and the District of Columbia.	No specific state data available	?	6a. Engage in collaborative study with key stakeholders on consumers' satisfaction with mental health services received in the regional catchment area. 6b. Study of state surveys done with 50 states including, District of Columbia and Puerto Rico. 49 out of 52 responded. Actual specific state results not available at this time (Survey of State Consumer Surveys, 2000).
7. Increase the number of States, Territories, and the District of Columbia with an operational mental health plan that addresses mental health crisis interventions, ongoing screening, and treatment services for elderly persons.	50 States and the District of Columbia.	No specific state data available	?	7a. Initiate direct contact with key stakeholders to ascertain the state specific operational mental health plan that addresses mental health crisis interventions, ongoing screening and treatment services for elderly persons in the regional catchment area. 7b. See 3b. 7c. Engage in further investigation for data with state representatives from the NASMHPD.

to the assessment team. Findings in which data was not readily available for assessment necessitated the proposal of specific recommendations. These recommendations require an additional commitment to data gathering and collaborative support with key stakeholders. Finally, any health care system or community group can promptly identify mental health and wellness needs and initiate steps to form recommendations to address the need(s) utilizing a comparison between the objective-related data and the *Healthy People 2010* target benchmarks.

 KEY POINTS

- Mental wellness is based on interconnected and dynamic states of total positive and negative energies arising from external and internal variables present within the eight subsystems of the community and directly from within the community.

- The inception of the deinstitutionalization movement paved the way for the current state of community-based services, including consumer-based mental health promotion and illness prevention activities.

- Issues central to legislation impacting mental health, such as parity and access to mental health services, can be tracked through developments within the federal government at http://thomas.loc.gov.

- A focus point, consistency, and collaborative approach to data collection that is agreed upon by key stakeholders of regional mental health agencies and services is essential to the needs assessment process.

- Resilience is a key contributing factor in predicting the overall mental health of individuals and in determining how individuals adapt and manage life stressors.

- Assessment of need requires recognition of cultural identities prevalent within the community and an understanding of the implications that influence residents' abilities to seek and respond to mental health services.

- Findings in which targeted data is not readily available for assessment against *Healthy People 2010* benchmarks necessitates further investigation and collaboration. The absence of data may demonstrate a crucial mental health need that is not being addressed. In addition, the discovery may influence the assessment team to refocus priorities and data gathering efforts.

◆ It is essential to seek a better understanding of resilience, its effectiveness, and its limits in reducing mental disorders and to build on this understanding to control risk factors.

REFERENCES

Alzheimer's disease: African-Americans at risk. (2001, July 30). *Nursing Spectrum, 14*(15IL), 5.

Alzheimer's Disease Education and Referral Center (ADEAR). (2001). Retrieved July 26, 20001, from National Institute on Aging: ADEAR. [Online]. Available: http://www.alzheimers.org/.

Alzheimer's disease menu. (2001). Retrieved July 26, 2001, from Massachusetts General Hospital, Department of Neurology WebForums. [Online]. Available: http://dem0nmac.mgh.harvard.edu/neurowebforum/AlzheimersDiseaseMenu.html.

Alzheimer's frequently discussed topics. (1995). Retrieved July 26, 2001, from Washington University in St. Louis, MO, Alzheimer's Disease Research Center. [Online]. Available: http://www.biostat.wustl.edu/alzheimer/frame1.html.

Alzheimer page. (2001). Retrieved July 26, 2001, from Washington University in St. Louis, MO, Alzheimer's Disease Research Center. [Online]. Available: http://www.biostat.wustl.edu/alzheimer/.

Alzheimer web home page. (2001). Retrieved July 26, 2001, from University of Melbourne, Department of Pathology. [Online]. Available: http://home.mira.net/~dhs/ad.html

American Psychiatric Association. (1994). *Diagnostic and statistical manual of mental disorders* (4th ed.). Washington, DC: Author.

Anderson, E., & McFarlane, J. (2000). *Community as partner* (4th ed.). Philadelphia: Lippincott.

Barry, M., Doherty, A., Hope, A., Sixsmith, J., & Kelleher, C. (2000). A community needs assessment for rural mental health promotion. *Health Education Research, 15*(3), 293–304.

Centers for Disease Control and Prevention. (1997). *Youth risk behavior surveillance—United States* (MMWR 47, No. SS-3). Atlanta, GA: Author.

Centers for Disease Control and Prevention. (2001). *Data 2010: . . . The Healthy People 2010 database.* [Online]. Available: http://www.health.gov./healthypeople/Data/data2010.htm.

Dementia Research Group. (1998). *Young onset dementia: Epidemiology, clinical symptoms, family burden, support and outcome.* [Online]. Available: http://dementia.ion.ucl.ac.uk/.

Dementia Research Group and CANDID (counseling and diagnosis in dementia). (2001). Retrieved July 26, 2001, from Dementia Research Group, Institute of Neurology. [Online]. Available: http://dementia.ion.ucl.ac.uk/.

Drug Prevention Resource Center. (2001). Retrieved July 27, 2001. [Online]. Available: http://www.drugs.indiana.edu/drug_stats/indiana.html

Epstein, M. H., Quinn, K., Cumblad, C., & Holderness, D. (1996). Needs assessment of community-based services for children and youth with emotional or behavioral disorders and their families: Part 1. A conceptual model. *Journal of Mental Health Administration, 23*(4), 418–431.

Fortinash, K., & Holoday-Worret, P. (2000). *Psychiatric mental health nursing* (2nd ed.). St. Louis, MO: Mosby.

Frisch, N., & Frisch, L. (1998). Psychiatric mental health nursing: Understanding the client as well as the condition. Clifton Park, NY: Delmar Learning.

Heale, J., & Abernathy, T. (1996). *Community health planning: Determining the needs of the community*. [Online]. Available: http://www.cwhpin.ca/.

Indiana Family and Social Services Administration (IFSSA) (2001). *Olmstead Data Collection Tool*. [Online]. Available: http://www.in.gov/fssa/servicedisabl/olmstead/olmsteaddata.html.

Indiana State Department of Health. (1999). *Indiana health behavior risk factors— 1998 state date (Appendix A: Healthy People 2000)*. [Online]. Available: http://www.in.gov/isdh/dataandstats/brfss/1998/app_a_table.htm.

Health Resources and Services Administration. (2000*). Community health status report: Lake County Indiana July 2000*. Merrifield, VA: U.S. Department of Health and Human Services.

IDEM and Public Health Subcommittee of the Environmental Quality Service Council. (1999, June). *Meeting minutes* (Meeting No. 3). Indianapolis, IN: Author.

Indiana Hospital Consumer Guide. (1996–1997). *Descriptions and selected data on the 50 most frequent APR-DRG's*. [Online]. Available: http://www.state.in.us/isdh/dataandstats/hospital/1996/table6–1.htm.

Indiana Alzheimer Disease Center (IADC) National Cell Repository. (2001). Retrieved February 20, 2001, from Indiana University School of Medicine, Department of Medical and Molecular Genetics. [Online]. Available: http://www.iupui.edu/~medgen/home2.html.

Kauffman, C., & Phillips, D. (2000). *Survey of state consumer surveys*. Rockville, MD: Survey and Analysis Branch Division of State and Community Systems Development Center for Mental Health Services Substance Abuse and Mental Health Services Administration.

Lake County Health Care Priorities. (1996). Indianapolis: Indiana State Department of Health.

Lee, R. H., Chamberlin, R., & Rapp, C. (2001). Brief report: System effects of the Kansas Mental Health Reform Act of 1991. *Community Mental Health Journal, 37*(5), 437–445.

Medicaid Intensive Community Mental Health Treatment Act of 2001, H.R. 2364, 107th Cong., 1st Sess. (2001). [Online]. Available: http://thomas.loc.gov/cgi-bin/query

Medicare Mental Health Modernization Act of 2001, S. 690, 107th Cong., 1st Sess. (2001). [Online]. Available: http://thomas.loc.gov/cgi-bin/query.

Mental Health Advisory Committee, H.R. Res. 14, 107th Cong., 1st Sess. (2001). [Online]. Available: http://thomas.loc.gov/cgi-bin/query/D?c107:36:./temp/~c107k4dUDN.

Mental Health and Substance Abuse Parity Amendments of 2001, H.R. 162, 107th Cong., 1st Sess. (2001). [Online]. Available: http://thomas.loc.gov/cgi-bin/query.

Mental Health Equitable Treatment Act of 2001, S. 543, 107th Cong., 1st Sess. Summary. (2001). [Online]. Available: http://thomas.loc.gov/cgi-bin/query.

National Institute of Mental Health. (2001). The impact of mental illness on society: . . . "The burden of psychiatric conditions has been heavily underestimated" [Online]. Available: http://www.nimh.nih.gov/publicat/burden.cfm.

Nardi, D., Sutherland, T., Tippy, F., Strupeck, D., et al. (2001). *Needs assessment of the health and wellbeing of Northwest Indiana.* Indiana University Northwest Shared Vision Research and Service Task Forces. Unpublished manuscript.

National Center for Chronic Disease Prevention and Health Promotion. (2000). *Youth Behavior Risk Surveys 1991, 1993,1995,1997, and 1999.* [Online]. Available: http://www.cdc.gov/nccdphp/dash/yrbs/trend.htm.

National Center for Health Statistics. (1999). *Healthy People 2000 review, 1998–1999: Mental health and mental disorders* (85–91) (DHHS Publication No. [PHS] 99–1256). [Online]. Available: http://www.cdc.gov/nchs/data/hp2k99.pdf.

National Center for Injury Prevention and Control. (2000). Retrieved July 27, 2001, from Injury Mortality Reports. [Online]. Available: http://webapp.cdc.gov/sasweb/ncipc/mortrate.html.

National Institute of Mental Health. (2001). *The numbers count: Mental disorders in America.* [Online]. Available: http://www.nimh.nih.gov/publicat/numbers.cfm

Physicians for a National Health Program: PNHP. (2000, September). *PHNP newsletter,* Chicago; IL: Author.

PRC Community Health Assessment. (1996). *Merrillville, Gary, Indiana.* Omaha, NE: Professional Research Consultants, Inc.

Quinn, K., Epstein, M. H., Cumblad, C., & Holderness, D. (1996). Needs assessment of community-based services for children and youth with emotional or behavioral disorders and their families: Part 2. Implementation in a local system of care. *Journal of Mental Health Administration, 23*(4), 432–446.

Royse, D., & Drude, K. (1995). Mental health needs assessment: Beware of false promises. *Community Mental Health Journal, 18*(2), 97–106.

Rural Mental Health Accessibility Act of 2001, S. 859, 107th Cong., 1st Sess, (2001). [Online]. Available: http://thomas.loc.gov/cgi-bin/query.

Schutt, R. (2001). *Investigating the social world* (3rd ed.). Boston: Pine Forge Press.

Silberner, J. (2001, July 5). To care for their child, they gave up custody. *All things considered.* National Public Radio, WNIB.

Spector, R. (2000). *Cultural care: Guides to heritage assessment and health traditions* (2nd ed.). Upper Saddle River, NJ: Prentice Hall Health.

Southlake Center for Mental Health Annual Report. (1999).

Stanhope, M., & Lancaster, J. (1996). *Community health nursing: Promoting health of aggregates, families, and individuals* (4th ed.). St. Louis, MO: Mosby.

Storandt, M., & Vandenbos, G. (Eds.). (1995*). Neuropsychological assessment of dementia and depression in older adults: A clinician's guide.* Washington, DC: American Psychological Association.

Stuart, G., & Laraia, M. (2001). *Principles and practices of psychiatric nursing* (7th ed.). St. Louis, MO: Mosby.

U.S. Department of Health and Human Services. (1995). *Healthy People 2000: Midcourse review and 1995 revisions* (pp. 53–57). [Online]. Available: http://odphp.osophs.dhhs.gov/pubs/hp2000/pdf/midcours/ch2–6.pdf.

U.S. Department of Health and Human Services. (1999). *Healthy People 2000 progress reviews: Mental health and mental disorders.* [Online]. Available: http://odphp.osophs.dhhs.gov/pubs/hp2000/PROG_RVW.HTM.

U.S. Department of Health and Human Services. (1999*). Mental health: A report of the Surgeon General.* Rockville, MD: U.S. Department of Health and Human Services, Substance Abuse and Mental Health Services Administration, Center for Mental Health Services, National Institute of Health, National Institute of Mental Health.

U.S. Department of Health and Human Services. (2000). *Healthy People 2010, volume II: Objectives for improving health (Part B: Focus areas 15–28)* (2nd ed.). [Online]. Available: http://www.health.gov./healthypeople/document/Word/volume2/18Mental.doc.

World Health Organization. (2001). *Definition of health.* [Online]. Available: www.who.int/aboutwho/en/definition.html

World Health Organization.(1999). Strengthening mental health promotion. [Online]. Available: http://www.who.int/inf-fs/en/fact220.html.

Chapter

5

ASSESSING MATERNAL, CHILD, AND FAMILY HEALTH AND WELLNESS

Deena A. Nardi
Debra Lugar

▬▬ LEARNING OBJECTIVES

At the conclusion of this chapter, the reader will be able to:

◆ Explore the physical, social, and environmental domains of maternal, child, and family health and wellness.

◆ Consider the impact of cultural variables on maternal, child, and family health.

◆ Identify a needs assessment problem related to maternal, child, and family health and well-being.

◆ Compare selected maternal, child, and family health and wellness indicators to *Healthy People 2010* benchmarks

◆ Construct a maternal, child, and family health and wellness needs assessment tool.

KEY TERMS

Early intervention	Prenatal
Fetal alcohol syndrome	Preterm
Folic acid	Social support
Full employment	Spina bifida
Low birth weight	Very low birth weight
Preconceptual planning	WIC

C hapter 5 demonstrates the use of the steps in the assessment of maternal, child, and family health and wellness. The health and wellness of children is assessed within the overall context of the functioning of the child-bearing family, including pregnancy planning, responsible sexual behaviors, maternal and infant care, and family health. Table 5-3 uses the *Healthy People 2010* goal of improving the health and well-being of women, infants, and families as an example of assessing the data and using it to guide planned interventions.

The health of pregnant and parenting women, the health and wellness of infants and children, and the well-being of families are key indicators of the quality of life of a community or neighborhood. They reflect not only the current health of the primary social unit of a country, but they are also predictive of the health of future generations. The social, physical, and environmental factors that impact maternal health and well-being affect the developing fetus either directly or indirectly. For instance, social factors such as the lifestyle choice of smoking during pregnancy or maternal stress level can affect developmental outcomes for children as well as quality of life outcomes for their families (Zuckerman, 1998).

Social factors include:

◆ Parenting style and caregiving

◆ Social support received during pregnancy and parenting

◆ Socioeconomic status (SES)

◆ Marital status

◆ Sexual activity and sexual responsibility, including intended pregnancies

◆ Lifestyle choices such as smoking or alcohol and drug use during pregnancy

PARENTING AND CAREGIVING

Ecological theory and the transactional model of child development are useful guides to understanding how social factors can impact a child's development. The basic premise of the transactional model of development is that outcomes are a product of the unique combination of an individual and what he or she experiences (Sameroff & Fiese, 1990). Urie Bronfenbrenner expands upon that premise in his ecological theory of human development by proposing that through an ongoing process of regulations, each child actively shapes and is influenced by his or her environment and own behavior (Bronfenbrenner, 1979). An ecological perspective on developmental risk looks inward to the child's responses (biologic and social) and outward to the social systems that shape the interactions of parent and child (Garbarino, 1990). This negotiative process is ever-changing, never static. As the growing child negotiates a changing world, both systems transform each other in a dialectical process of development (Riegel, 1975). In other words, developing children influence their families, families influence the development of their children, and both are influenced by their communities, as their communities are also shaped by the health of their families.

At birth, a child brings to his or her personal experience a full complement of genes that have determined eye color, height, gender, maturity of nervous system response, and possibly temperament (the quality and adjustment of response in an individual that cannot be explained by learned behavior theory). This genotype, or biological organization, also accounts for physical handicaps, disorders of emotional and nervous system regulation due to perinatal drug exposure, learning disabilities, and susceptibility to certain psychopathologic disorders such as schizophrenia or bipolar disorder.

This genotype will influence a child's responses to moment-to-moment interactions with parents, to caregiving regulations, and to major changes of experience that occur as the child develops. These include the beginning of toilet training, parallel play and school, and changes in the exosystem (for example, parents lose, change, or begin jobs, or the family SES changes).

Concurrently, the moment-to-moment parental attachment behaviors and the personal working models that guide parental responses also affect a child's biological organization (e.g., a soothing voice and swaddling can calm a colic attack). This transactional duet between parent and child places both responses in an active dialectic that transforms both. This transactional dance occurs in a wider social system (the environtype in transactional theory and the exosystem in ecologic theory) and is also influenced by the participants, cultural expectations, social laws, and economic forces that shape the parents' caregiving regulations and the child's developing regulations (Fiese & Sameroff, 1989; Sameroff & Fiese, 1990; Garbarino, 1990; Bronfenbrenner, 1990). *Healthy People 2010* goal 16, objective 19, "Increase proportion of mothers who breastfeed their babies to 75%," provides benchmarks that can be used for this health and wellness outcome (U.S. Department of Health and Human Services, 2000).

SOCIAL SUPPORT

Social support is another factor that impacts a child's development. It has been included in a number of studies on parenting among groups at higher risk for poor developmental outcomes. **Social support** is the feeling of being cared for by others. It can be divided into three components: nurturance, recognition, and group membership. It can be both qualitative and quantitative in nature, and has the following properties: *interactional properties*—which contain content, intensity, and frequency components; *social network properties*—which contain range, consistency, accessibility, and affiliative components; *subjective properties*—which contain one's perceptions of being supported and giving support (Pearson, 1986). It is complex and multifaceted, and operates concurrently with other factors, such as level of SES, parenting behaviors, and lifestyle (Nath, Whitman, Borkowski, & Schellenbach, 1990). Social support can buffer the effects of stress on parenting (Unger & Wasserman, 1988), and is related to more positive health outcomes (Nath, Whitman, Borkowski, & Schellenbach, 1990). However, types of social support might also yield different outcomes depending on other factors, such as age, SES, individual perception, and needs. If the effect of social support in all its forms and classifications is transactional, and not simply cumulative or direct in nature, this might account for the negative outcomes that have also been associated with social support.

The extended family is viewed as a significant source of social support for many cultural groups in the United States. However, it has a dual nature, causing negative as well as positive effects on family life. For instance, if community supportive network services for the African American family aren't individualized to meet the mother's needs, they can lead to a feeling of loss of personal control, so important to self-esteem. Boyd-Franklin (1987) noted that "many black women feel so absorbed by duties and responsibilities in the nuclear family that they have little emotional energy left for themselves. This pattern, once established within the family of origin, can be repeated in countless new relationships unless it is checked and changed" (p. 398). Miller (1988) notes that several studies of family support for Black families show an inverse relationship between this extended family support and the recipient's self-esteem. *Healthy People 2010* goal 16, objective 19, "Increase proportion of States that have service systems for children with special health care needs to 100%," provides benchmarks that can be used for this health and wellness outcome (U.S. Department of Health and Human Services, 2000).

SOCIOECONOMIC AND MARITAL STATUS

Socioeconomic status is a major determinant of maternal and child health, since it impacts all of the other determinants, such as quality of schools, access to quality health care, safe housing, and even proper nutrition (Adler, Boyce, Chesney, Cohen, Folkman, Kahn, & Syme, 1994; Nelson, 1994). For instance, life expectancies are related to socioeconomic status, with those in a higher socioeconomic level living longer (Kochanek, Maurer, & Rosenberg, 1994). Families who are poor, or who live in counties with poverty-level or below standard of living, are more vulnerable to poor health outcomes, such as higher infant and child death rates, acquired immunodeficiency syndrome, and diabetes (Hamburg, 1998). They experience disparities in access to health care, and their health outcomes are comparable to those in Third World countries (NRHA, 1999). However, the benefits related to socioeconomic status might be due to the secondary benefits of the greater financial resources available, which offer more lifestyle choices and options, and permit healthier lifestyles, better nutrition, access to affordable health care and even stress reduction through vacations. *Healthy People 2010* goal 17, objective 1, "Increase high school completion," provides benchmarks that can be used for this health and wellness outcome (U.S. Department of Health and Human Services, 2000).

Marital status has been linked to health outcomes for all age groups. Several studies have demonstrated the positive relationship between a happy marriage and emotional and physical well-being in children (Dawson, 1991; Gottman & Katz, 1989). Even birth outcomes, such as normal birth weights, are more positive for married couples (Donovan & Sanders, 1999). The protective factors provided by marriage probably include the advantage of an additional or full-time income, added social support, and increased emotional well-being. *Healthy People 2010* goal 7, objective 3, "Increase the proportion of college and universities students who receive information from their institution on each of the six priority health-risk behavior areas," provides benchmarks that can be used for this health and wellness outcome (U.S. Department of Health and Human Services, 2000).

SEXUAL ACTIVITY AND SEXUAL RESPONSIBILITY, INCLUDING INTENDED PREGNANCIES

Healthy People 2010 goals for responsible sexual behaviors, including family planning, are largely based on the findings from the 1995 Institute of Medicine report (Brown & Eisenberg, 1995). This report states that 60 percent of all pregnancies are unintended, and echoes findings of other studies: women carrying unintended pregnancies to term are more likely to postpone prenatal care (Kost, Landry, & Darroch, 1998); their newborns are more likely to be low birthweight; the mother is more likely to have a history of sexual abuse (Stock, Bell, Boyer, & Connell, 1997). The report emphasizes that healthy lifestyles by both men and women, including preconceptual planning, ensures healthy families.

Preconceptual planning is a process of actively planning for conception, pregnancy, and birth, incorporating the three components of health promotion, risk assessment, and proper treatment (WAPC, 2000). Health promotion activities would include providing counseling and education about reducing risks to a healthy pregnancy, and assessing for the presence of social and emotional support and access to perinatal care. Risk assessment would include conducting a complete physical exam, obtaining a thorough health and psychosocial history from both parents, and conducting appropriate laboratory tests. Laboratory tests should include screening for HIV and other sexually transmitted diseases (STDs), which are linked to unprotected sexual behaviors (Brunham, Holmes, & Embree, 1990). STDs increase the risk of infant death or disease, since STDs can cross the placenta and infect the fetus (Goldenberg, Andrews, Yuan, MacKay, et al., 1997). Proper treatment would include instituting a multivitamin regimen, which would include folic acid, appropriate contraception or infertility treatment if needed, and other specialty care if needed, such as diabetes treatment or genetic testing. *Healthy People 2010* goal 9, objective 1, "Improve pregnancy planning and spacing and prevent unintended pregnancy," provides benchmarks that can be used for this health and wellness outcome (U.S. Department of Health and Human Services, 2000).

LIFESTYLE CHOICES

Maternal smoking begins as a lifestyle choice and becomes a habit on its way to an addiction, and in the process can cause physical harm to the mother and impede fetal development. Health effects to the mother include acute and chronic bronchitis, emphysema, chronic obstructive lung disease, cardiovascular disease, cancer, osteoporosis, and periodontal disease (National Heart, Lung, and Blood Institute, 1995).

There is growing concern about the reported increase in the number of infants born to mothers who are using controlled substances and psychoactive drugs and alcohol during pregnancy. Maternal drug abuse and alcohol use is a major risk factor for newborn developmental disabilities, learning disorders, low birth weight and death (Camas, Cheung & Lieberman, 1995; Stratton, Howe, & Battaglia, 1996). *Healthy People 2010* goal 16, objective 17, "Increase abstinence from alcohol, cigarettes, and other illicit drugs among pregnant women to 94%," provides benchmarks that can be used for these health and wellness outcomes (U.S. Department of Health and Human Services, 2000).

Smoking during pregnancy is also a major risk factor for low birth weight and preterm births. **Low birth weight** (LBW) refers to a newborn that weighs less than 2500 grams (5.5 pounds) at birth. LBW and preterm births account for 20 percent of newborn deaths (Ventura, Martin, Curtin, & Mathews, 1999). **Preterm** birth is one occurring before the 37th week of gestation. These factors also increase risk for neonatal death or developmental disabilities such as vision and hearing impairment, learning disabilities, cerebral palsy, and even infantile autism (Ventura, Martin, Curtin, & Mathews, 1999; Hoyert, 1996). Included in these findings are neonates of **very low birth weight.** Very low birth weight (VLBW) refers to infants who weigh less than 1500 grams (3 pounds) at birth. *Healthy People 2010* goal 16, objective 11, "Reduce preterm births to 7.6%," and objective 10, "Reduce low birth weight and very low birth weight to 5.0% for low birth weight and 0.9% for very low birth weight," provides benchmarks that can be used for these health and wellness outcomes (U.S. Department of Health and Human Services, 2000).

Physical factors that impact maternal child and family health and wellness include:

◆ Proper prenatal care and maternal nutrition

◆ Breastfeeding

◆ Maternal tobacco, drug, and alcohol use before and during pregnancy

◆ Chronic illnesses and disabilities of children

PROPER PRENATAL CARE AND MATERNAL NUTRITION

Proper prenatal care lowers the risk for low and very low birth weights, fetal alcohol syndrome, neural tube defects such as spina bifida, and preterm births (Grad & Hill, 1992). **Prenatal** refers to the period of time from conception to labor, when a woman is pregnant and the child is developing in the womb. Studies show repeatedly that quality prenatal care can prevent many of the developmental disorders and family situations that place children and their families at risk for violence, abuse, poor school performance, and poverty. Proper prenatal care includes preconception screening for genetic disorders, assessment and counseling to identify and minimize the effects of social, physical, and environmental risk factors affecting the mother, a vitamin regimen started as early as possible in the pregnancy and continuing throughout the pregnancy, regularly scheduled physicals, abstaining from drugs and alcohol, proper nutrition, and enrollment in WIC, if indicated (U.S. Department of Health and Human Services, 2000). **WIC** is an acronym for the Women, Infants and Children program, a federally funded, state-administered food assistance program offering nutrition assistance to low-income pregnant and breastfeeding women, infants, and children up to age 5.

Nutrition and vitamin supplements should include daily **folic acid,** which is a protective factor against the development of neural tube defects such as spina bifida in the fetus (Boyle & Zola, 1996). **Spina bifida** is a congenital defect at the lower end of the spinal column, or a neural tube defect, which may result in varying degrees of physical impairment that can include paralysis below the waist with loss of bowel and bladder control. *Healthy People 2010* goal 16, objective 6, "Increase proportion of pregnant women who receive early and adequate prenatal care to 90% in first trimester, and 90% receiving early and adequate care," and objective 7, "Increase proportion of pregnant women who attend a series of prepared childbirth classes," provide benchmarks that can be used for these health and wellness outcomes (U.S. Department of Health and Human Services, 2000).

BREASTFEEDING

The practice of breastfeeding improves the quality of life for newborns, their mothers, and their families. It reduces infection rate in the newborn (Beaudry, Dufour & Marcoux, 1995) and can improve the health and even the economic status of the new mother (Dewey, Heinig, & Nommsen, 1993; Montgomery & Splett, 1997). Although the practice of breastfeeding has been increasing in recent years, rates are still very low. Rates of breastfeeding in 1997 at five and six months after birth were 29 percent for Caucasian Americans, 24.5 percent for Hispanics, and 14.5 percent for African Americans (Mothers' Survey, 1998). These rates call for assessment of plans to breastfeed at a prenatal screening, and breastfeeding instruction and support services such as lactation counseling that are culturally appropriate and targeted to specific cultural groups. *Healthy People 2010* goal 16, objective 19, "Increase proportion of mothers who breastfeed their babies to 75%," provides benchmarks that can be used for this health and wellness outcome (U.S. Department of Health and Human Services, 2000).

MATERNAL TOBACCO, DRUG, AND ALCOHOL USE BEFORE AND DURING PREGNANCY

Although maternal tobacco drug and alcohol use before and during pregnancy has been addressed in an earlier section under "lifestyle choice," the use of these substances during pregnancy deserves special attention, because of their links to infant death, low birth weight, mental retardation, and fetal alcohol syndrome (FAS) (Zuckerman, 1998; Jones, 1986). FAS is an especially grievous developmental disability because it is completely preventable if the mother does not use alcohol while pregnant. **Fetal alcohol syndrome** (FAS) is a birth defect of infants whose mothers consume alcohol during pregnancy. Effects on the infant include mental retardation, behavior and growth problems, structural abnormalities of the face and limbs, and other abnormalities. The degree of involvement is related to the amount of alcohol consumed and the duration and pregnancy stage in which it occurred. No specific amount of alcohol is known to be a cause, hence abstinence during pregnancy is recommended. Diagnosis is based upon the detection of three hallmarks: perinatal growth retardation, central nervous system impairment, and certain characteristic facial abnormalities (Lundsberg, Bracken, & Saftlas, 1997; American Academy of Pediatrics, 1995). *Healthy People 2010,* goal 16, objective 18, "Reduce the occurrence of fetal alcohol syndrome (FAS)," provides benchmarks that can be used for these health and wellness outcomes (U.S. Department of Health and Human Services, 2000).

CHRONIC ILLNESSES AND DISABILITIES OF CHILDREN

The health of children affects their school readiness, or ability to learn in school (Riley & Shalala, 1994). Because children with chronic illnesses or disabilities are at risk for developmental disability or delay, federal legislation has been passed to provide coordinated delivery of early intervention services from infancy to age 18, to address their special health care needs, and to prevent or minimize any developmental disabilities (Ruppert, 1997). The federal definition of a developmental disability (DD) is contained in the Developmental Disabilities Assistance and Bill of Rights

Act of 1990, Public Law 101-496, Section 102. It defines DD as a severe or chronic disability of individuals ages 5 to 22, due to a mental or physical impairment or combination of both, that will continue indefinitely and can result in substantive limitation in three or more of the following domains: learning, language, mobility, independent living, economic self-sufficiency, self-care, and self-direction. This term is also applied to children ages newborn to 5, who demonstrate substantial developmental delay, have special congenital conditions, or have acquired conditions that indicate a high risk for developmental disability.

Early intervention is a coordinated system of services for infants and toddlers who have or are at risk for developmental disabilities, designed to prevent or minimize the disability to the degree possible. All children with chronic illnesses or disabilities should be receiving condition-appropriate early intervention services if they are age 5 or under, or free-appropriate public education and supportive services as needed when older. These services should be community-based and culturally competent, and should include screening, regular assessment, family support, consistent caregivers, special instruction if warranted, counseling for the child, and family and case management services (American Academy of Pediatrics, 1999; Wallace & Gittler, 1998).

Healthy People 2010, objective 16–14, "reduce the occurrence of developmental disabilities," has targeted the four developmental disability groupings of mental retardation, cerebral palsy, autism spectrum disorder, and epilepsy for specific reduction in rate by the year 2010 (U.S. Department of Health and Human Services, 2000). Every community should have provisions for early intervention, public education and support services available for their children and families with special needs. *Healthy People 2010,* goal 16, objective 22, "Increase the proportion of children with special health care needs who have access to a medical home," provides benchmarks that can be used for these health and wellness outcomes (U.S. Department of Health and Human Services, 2000).

Environmental factors include:

◆ Neighborhood and community violence

◆ Access to quality schools

◆ Employment opportunities

NEIGHBORHOOD AND COMMUNITY VIOLENCE

Interpersonal violence is a major public health problem, and is recognized as such by the World Health Organization (World Health Assembly, 1996; Foege, Rosenberg, & Mercy, 1995). Homicide is the second leading cause of death among adults ages 15 to 24 in the United States, and the first cause of death among African Americans in this age group (Singh, Kochanek, & Mac Dorman, 1994). The overwhelming majority of perpetrators of child maltreatment are the parents of the victims (HHS, 1997); other forms of domestic violence such as intimate partner abuse are considered family violence. Family violence has far-reaching effects on the well-being of family members and the safety and livability of the neighborhood or community (Kent-Wilkerson, 1996). *Healthy People 2010,* goal 16, objective 34, "Reduce the rate of physical assault by current or former intimate partners," provides one of the benchmarks that can be used for these health and wellness outcomes (U.S. Department of Health and Human Services, 2000).

ACCESS TO QUALITY SCHOOLS

High school completion decreases the risk for unemployment, poverty, poor health, and a number of related social problems such as substance abuse, abuse and violence, and family dysfunction (Palfrey, 1995; Schorr, 1989). The U.S. Department of Education (1991) has made access to quality schools its number one priority because of the importance of high school completion to quality of life for individuals and their communities (National Education Goals Panel, 1999). Any assessment of community maternal child and family health should include high school completion rates and adult literacy levels. Additional information would include class sizes, college graduation rates, and number and types of adjunct and social services programs (such as art classes and school lunches), available in the public school system. *Healthy People 2010,* goal 7, objective 1, "Increase high school completion," provides one of the benchmarks that can be used for these health and wellness outcomes (U.S. Department of Health and Human Services, 2000).

EMPLOYMENT OPPORTUNITIES

Full employment improves the health of the community both directly and indirectly. **Full employment** means that the worker is employed full-time, or 40 hours per week, with customary benefits such as individual and family health insurance and vacation/illness pay (Centers for Disease Control and Prevention, 1995). Access to quality health services is a *Healthy People 2010* focus area, since the primary and preventative services this access provides will improve quality of life, increase the number of healthy days, and decrease health disparities from race, ethnicity, SES group, or location (Reinhardt, 1994; U.S. General Accounting Office, 1998). Employment opportunities in the community also provide a sense of hope for the future, which is in itself a preventative from gang-related activity and abusive behavior. *Healthy People 2010,* goal 1, objective 1, "Increase the proportion of persons with health insurance," provides one of the benchmarks that can be used for these health and wellness outcomes (U.S. Department of Health and Human Services, 2000).

STEPS OF ASSESSING MATERNAL, CHILD, AND FAMILY HEALTH AND WELLNESS

Six goals of *Healthy People 2010* addressing the assessment and functioning of the health and wellness of families are presented in this chapter. These goals were selected for their overall interrelationship and impact upon the safety and security of children, their parents, and the overall functioning of their families. Goals involving pregnancy planning (9), HIV prevention (13), and responsible sexual behaviors (25), all have as their common focus the safe conception, development, and delivery of healthy infants to families that are equipped to safeguard and care for them. Goals involving vaccinations (14), improve the health of women, infants, and families (16), and safe use of medical products (17), have as their common focus the maintenance of the health of these families. Table 5-1 presents these six goals, the general topics or issues they address, and their relationship to related *Healthy People 2010* goals and objectives.

Step One: Defining and Describing the Purpose of a Community Needs Assessment Related to Maternal, Child, and Family Health And Wellness

The assessment of the needs of maternal, child, and family health focuses primarily on pregnant and parenting women, mothers, infants, children, and their families and the issues that affect their health directly and indirectly. Although males are part of the family unit, the physical and mental health needs of males are not addressed in *Healthy People 2010* goal 16, which was chosen as this chapter's example. The health needs of males are addressed in the goals discussed in Chapters 3 and 4.

When identifying the need for a health assessment, the assessment team must decide what part of the family unit will be included, as this will determine not only the *Healthy People 2010* goals chosen as benchmarks, but will determine what data is collected and which sources are used. In

TABLE 5-1 *Healthy People 2010 Maternal, Child, and Families Goals*

GOAL #	GENERAL TOPIC	HEALTHY PEOPLE 2010 GOAL	RELATED HEALTHY PEOPLE 2010 GOALS & OBJECTIVES
9	Family planning	Improve pregnancy planning and spacing and prevent unintended pregnancy.	*HIV* 13-6. Condom use *Maternal deaths and illnesses* 16-4. Maternal deaths 16-5. Maternal illnesses and complications due to pregnancy *Prenatal care* 16-6. Prenatal care 16-7. Childbirth classes *Risk factors* 16-12. Weight gain during pregnancy *Prenatal substance exposure* 16-17. Prenatal substance exposure 16-18. Fetal alcohol syndrome *Personal health* 25-17. Screening of pregnant women
13	HIV	Prevent HIV infection and it's related illness and death.	*Family planning* 9-3. Contraceptive use 9-8. Abstinence before age 15 9-9. Abstinence among adolescents aged 15–17 years *Universal precautions* 14-3. Hepatitis B in adults and high risk groups

continues

TABLE 5-1 *Healthy People 2010* Maternal, Child, and Families Goals *continued*

GOAL #	GENERAL TOPIC	HEALTHY PEOPLE 2010 GOAL	RELATED HEALTHY PEOPLE 2010 GOALS & OBJECTIVES
14	Immunizations & infectious diseases	Prevent disease, disability, and death from infectious diseases, including vaccine preventable diseases.	*Vaccination coverage* 14–28. Hepatitis B vaccination among high risk groups *Family planning* 9–12. Problems becoming pregnant and maintaining a pregnancy *HIV* 13–5. New HIV cases 13–13. Treatment according to guidelines 13–14. HIV infection deaths 13–17. Perinatally acquired HIV infection *Childhood deaths* 16–1. Fetal and infant deaths 16–2. Child deaths 16–3. Adolescent and young adult deaths *Risk factors* 16–10. Low birth weight and very low birth weight 16–11. Preterm births *Breast feeding, newborn screening and service systems* 16–21. Sepsis among children with sickle cell disease 16–22. Medical homes for children with special health care needs 16–23. Service systems for children with special health care needs

| 16 | Women and children's health | Improve health and well being of women, infants, and families. | *Bacterial STD illness*
25-1. Chlamydia
25-2. Gonorrhea
25-3. Primary and secondary syphilis
Viral STD illness
25-4. Genital herpes
STD complications in females
25-8. Heterosexually transmitted HIV infection in women
Community protection infrastructure
25-13. Hepatitis B vaccine services in STD clinics
25-14. Screening youth detention facilities and jails
25-15. Contracts to treat non-plan partners of STD patients

Family planning
9-1. Intended pregnancies
9-2. Birth spacing
9-3. Contraceptive use
9-6. Male involvement in pregnancy prevention
9-8. Abstinence before age 15
9-9. Abstinence among adolescents aged 15–17 years
HIV
13-7. Knowledge of serostatus
13-12. Screening for STDs and immunization for hepatitis B
13-13. Treatment according to guidelines
13-17. Perinatally acquired HIV infection |

continues

TABLE 5-1   *Healthy People 2010 Maternal, Child, and Families Goals* *continued*

GOAL #	GENERAL TOPIC	HEALTHY PEOPLE 2010 GOAL	RELATED HEALTHY PEOPLE 2010 GOALS & OBJECTIVES
			Universal precautions 14-1. Vaccine preventable diseases 14-2. Hepatitis B in infants and young children 14-3. Hepatitis B among adults and high risk groups 14-4. Bacterial meningitis in young children *Infectious diseases* 14-18. Antibiotics prescribed for ear infections 14-19. Antibiotics prescribed for common cold *Vaccination coverage* 14-22. Universally recommended vaccinations of children aged 19–35 months 14-23. Vaccination coverage for children in day care, kindergarten and first grade 14-24. Fully immunized young children and adolescents 14-25. Providers who measure childhood vaccination coverage levels *Safe medical products* 17-3. Provider review of medications taken by patients 17-4. Receipt of useful information about prescriptions from pharmacies 17-5. Receipt of oral counseling about medications from prescribers and dispensers

STD complications affecting females
25-7. Fertility problems
25-8. Heterosexually transmitted HIV infection in women
STD complications affecting the fetus and newborn
25-9. Congenital syphilis
25-10. Neonatal STDs
Personal behaviors
25-11. Responsible adolescent sexual behavior
25-12. Responsible sexual behavior messages on television
Personal health services
25-16. Annual screening for chlamydia
25-17. Screening of pregnant women
25-18. Compliance with recognized STD treatment guidelines
25-19. Provider services for sex partners

Family planning
9-4 Contraceptive failure
9-10. Pregnancy protection and sexually transmitted disease prevention
HIV
13-6. Condom use
Vaccine safety
14-30. Adverse events from vaccinations
14-31. Active surveillance for vaccine safety
Breast feeding, newborn screening and service systems
16-20. Newborn bloodspot screening

| 17 | Safe medical products | Ensure the safe and effective use of medical products. |

continues

TABLE 5-1   *Healthy People 2010 Maternal, Child, and Families Goals* continued

GOAL #	GENERAL TOPIC	HEALTHY PEOPLE 2010 GOAL	RELATED HEALTHY PEOPLE 2010 GOALS & OBJECTIVES
25	Responsible sexual behavior	Promote responsible sexual behaviors, strengthen communities capacity, and increase quality services to prevent sexually transmitted diseases and their complications.	*Family planning*
			9–1. Intended pregnancies
			9–2. Birth spacing
			9–3. Contraceptive use
			9–4. Emergency contraceptive use
			9–8. Abstinence before age 15
			9–9. Abstinence among adolescents aged 15–17 years
			9–10. Pregnancy prevention and sexually transmitted disease protection
			9–11. Pregnancy prevention education
			HIV
			13–6. Condom use
			13–13. Treatment according to guidelines
			13–17. Perinatally acquired HIV infection
			Vaccinations coverage
			14–3. Hepatitis B in adults and high risk groups
			14–28. Hepatitis B vaccination among high risk groups
			Prenatal care
			16–6. Prenatal care
			Prenatal substance exposure
			16–17. Prenatal substance exposure

Source: Reprinted with permission from the Department of Health and Human Services. (January, 2000). *Healthy people 2010.* Conference Edition, in Two Volumes). Washington, DC.

determining the purpose of the maternal child and family health assessment, the team must also choose a target population. In the community health and wellness assessment done by Nardi et al. (2000), a tri-county region was chosen, but the assessment team had to decide what geographic area best suited their stated needs. In the three county areas used in their assessment, the population was an ethnic mix of Caucasian, African American, and Hispanic with other smaller, minority groups. Table 5-2 lists the proportion of distinct ethnic populations in the area. After reviewing the U.S. Census data regarding the area, the team decided that the tri-county area would adequately represent the ethnic diversity of the larger region.

Step Two: Choosing *Healthy People 2010* Goals and Benchmarks

When beginning a maternal, child, and family health and wellness needs assessment, the assessment team must select the *Healthy People 2010* goals that will be utilized, so that the data collected will reflect areas included in each goal. For example, if the goal is to improve the safety of children, the goals could address physical safety (seat belt use, violence), safety related to medication usage (correct administration, storage of medication), or safety from infection (immunizations). Objectives must be derived from these goals, and used to guide choice of resources and information gathered.

The benchmarks selected to be used in the assessment of the health and well-being needs of women, infants, children, and families might relate to those that most closely affect the unity of the family and its development over a life span from dyad to triad. Families are composed of parents and children but may also include grandparents, aunts, uncles, and cousins (extended family). The health of each member of a family can affect the health and well-being of the entire unit as well as the extended members. For example, some illnesses such as HIV can have long-term impacts on families socially and economically in addition to the basic

TABLE 5-2   Ethnic Makeup Reported in 2000 U.S. Census

ETHNIC GROUP	LAKE COUNTY, INDIANA	INDIANA
White persons	66.7%	87.5%
Black or African American	25.3%	8.4%
Hispanic or Latino *	12.2%	3.5%

*May be of any race and are included in other race categories.

health concerns associated with the disease process. Many health care providers do not consider HIV infection as a possible diagnosis in young child-bearing women and as a result, females tend to be diagnosed with HIV infections later than males (Harkey, 1997). This late diagnosis contributes to poorer outcomes and affects the entire family unit.

Individuals or groups planning a needs assessment focusing on the health and well-being of women, children, and families might choose the same *Healthy People 2010* goals and benchmarks as those chosen by the regional assessment team used as an example throughout this chapter.

Step Three: Information Gathering

Data can be collected from various sources. No one way of data collection will be effective in all communities. In the example used throughout this text, data is derived from a regional needs assessment conducted at a local university (Nardi et al., 2000). Sources include public university libraries, Internet sites, and conversations with local Health Departments and hospitals. In this instance students enrolled in a community health course conducted a community assessment and provided some data for the regional health and well-being needs assessment. Reports of this nature are not generally published; indeed, many hospitals and local government agencies may conduct similar surveys that are not published. This makes contacting such organizations imperative to a comprehensive community assessment. The remainder of this section presents the nuances of the six goals from *Healthy People 2010* that correspond to maternal, child, and family health and wellness. An example of the use of resources to assess one goal illustrates the use of secondary data sources to gather pertinent data.

Goal Nine: Pregnancy Planning

Goal 9 is "Improve pregnancy planning and spacing and prevent unintended pregnancies." The objectives for goal 9 address family planning from the aspect of planned and unplanned pregnancies as well as various contraceptives available. An association is made between the risk of pregnancy and the risk of sexually transmitted diseases (STDs). Also of concern to the health of the family is promoting abstinence for those under age 17 and male involvement in the prevention of pregnancies. An example of achievement of this goal would be to have insurance coverage for contraceptive supplies and services.

Goal Thirteen: HIV Prevention

Goal 13 is "Prevent HIV infection and its related illness and death." The number of persons who are HIV positive is on the rise. Females with HIV may pass the virus to their unborn offspring, thereby causing the number of children affected to be on the rise also. This goal addresses the prevention, diagnosis, counseling, treatment, and education for families as well as risk factors associated with transmission of HIV.

Goal Fourteen: Vaccinations

Goal 14 is "Prevent disease, disability, and death from infectious diseases, including vaccine-preventable diseases." Many childhood diseases are preventable with proper immunization, yet there are children who do not receive proper immunizations by school age. Goal 14 addresses the need to immunize children against various infectious diseases and includes recommended immunization schedules. Also of concern is the increase in the spread of tuberculosis (TB), and its diagnosis and therapy are discussed.

Goal Sixteen: Improve Health of Women, Infants, and Families

Goal 16 is "Improve the health and well being of women, infants, children, and families." Improving the health of women and infants is directly related to a woman's health status during pregnancy. By increasing the number of pregnant women who seek early prenatal care, it is hoped the community will see a decrease in the number of pregnancies that have complications and thereby fewer incidences of children with long-term disabilities.

Goal Seventeen: Safe Use of Medical Products

Goal 17 is "Ensure the safe and effective use of medical products." Medical products are primarily medications and include printed information dispensed with prescriptions as well as verbal instructions and counseling given by pharmacies. Monitoring adverse medical events and blood transfusions are also addressed.

Goal Twenty-Five: Responsible Sexual Behaviors

Goal 25 is "Promote responsible sexual behaviors, strengthen community capacity, and increase access to quality services to prevent sexually transmitted diseases (STDs) and their complications." This goal addresses various STDs in regard to disability and complications such as infertility. In addition, of concern are the complications caused by transmission to a fetus or newborn infant. Screening for STDs in clinics, jails, and among pregnant females as well as notifications of sex partners is addressed.

Some examples of resources for gathering data might include the secondary analysis of existing data from the following:

◆ Infant mortality rate (Health Resources, 2000)

◆ Prenatal care data (Indiana Natality, 2000)

◆ Very low birth weight, low birth weight, and pre-term birth data (Indiana Natality, 2000)

◆ Use of alcohol, tobacco, and illicit drugs during pregnancy data (Indiana Natality, 2000)

◆ Data on the proportion of women discharged from hospitals breastfeeding (Indiana Natality, 2000)

◆ Pregnancy Risk Assessment Monitoring System (PRAMS) data (Centers for Disease Control, Reproductive Health, 2000)

Focus groups might be conducted at the following sites:

◆ Local area hospitals and clinics

◆ Local elementary and high schools, colleges, universities, and churches

◆ Legislators

Key informants can be solicited from the following groups:

◆ Practitioners involved in drug rehabilitation programs

◆ Local physicians, nurse practitioners, midwives, childbirth educators, lactation consultants

◆ Participants in nutrition programs, including WIC

◆ Professionals involved with rehab programs and addiction counselors

◆ Providers of child care and immunization clinics

◆ Participants in PRAMS

Step Four: Analysis of the Information

The following data is an example of the type of information that was gathered by the assessment team during their assessment of maternal child and family health and wellness indicators:

◆ In one county, the infant mortality rate from 1995 to 1997 was 10.3, the White infant mortality rate was 6.9, the Black infant mortality rate was 17.7, the neonatal infant mortality rate was 7.0, and the post-natal infant mortality rate was 3.3. All rates indicate a status less than favorable (Health Resources, 2000).

◆ In one county, the percent of infants born with low birth weight (< 2500 g) was 8.7 percent, compared to the *Healthy People 2010* target of 5.0 percent. Percentage of very low birth rates (< 1500 g) was 1.7 percent, compared to the *Healthy People 2010* target of 0.9 percent. Percentage of premature births (< 37 weeks) was 12.8 percent compared to the *Healthy People 2010* target of 7.6 percent. 46.2% births were to unmarried women. 24.2 percent of newborns had no prenatal care in the first trimester, compared to the *Healthy People* target of 10.0 percent (Health Resources, 2000).

◆ The state did not belong to PRAMS, the Pregnancy Risk Assessment Monitoring System, a surveillance project of the Centers for Disease Control and Prevention and state Health Departments. PRAMS provides data for state health officials to use to improve the health of mothers and infants. Its purpose is to improve the health of mothers and infants by reducing adverse birth outcomes (Centers for Disease Control, Reproductive Health, 2000).

◆ In 1997, the teen birth rate was 37.6 percent for one county, 32.1 percent in another county, and 18.1 percent in a third county, and 32.1 percent in the state (Heartland Center, 2000).

◆ Obstetrical-related admitting diagnoses were the top-ranked DRGs for inpatient care for Methodist hospitals for 1999 (C. Biancardi, Methodist Hospitals, personal communication, October 23, 2000).

This collection of data had little meaning until it was placed in the assessment tool. Table 5-3 presents the results of the assessment of maternal child and family health and wellness related to *Healthy People 2010* goal 16, categorized by that goal's 23 objectives as benchmarks in the first column, which could be compared to the collected data in the second column. The third column identifies if there is a need, and the fourth column is used to consider recommendations for intervention.

The data concerning this one goal indicates that not all relevant *Healthy People 2010* objectives have been met, either because a need was clearly indicated or because the indicated data was not readily available to the assessment team. By using the needs assessment tool a comparison between the objective-related data and the target benchmarks assisted the assessment team in readily identifying health and wellness needs in this area and taking steps to form recommendations to address the need.

TABLE 5-3 Needs Assessment: Maternal, Child, and Family Health and Wellness

GOAL 16: Improve Health and Well-Being of Women, Infants and Families.

HP 2010 OBJECTIVES	TARGET	DATA ASSESSED	NEED	RECOMMENDATIONS
1. Reduction in infant deaths related to birth defects.	Reduce to 4.1 per 1000 live births ∃ 20 wks gestation; 4.5 per 1000 in perinatal period; 4.5 per 1000 for all infants per year; reduce SIDS deaths to 0.3 per 1000.	In 1995–1997 in Lake County, the infant mortality rate was 10.3 for white infants, 17.7 for blacks infants; the neonatal mortality rate was 7.0 and the post natal mortality rate was 3.3 (Health Resources, 2000).	X	Develop a regional health and wellness center, affiliated with area hospitals, to meet primary health needs of pregnant women, infants and children who are underserved.
2. Reduce the rate of child deaths.	Reduce to 25 per 1000 for 1–4 yr olds; 14.3 per 1000 for 5–9 yr olds.	No data	?	Identify common causes of death among children in the target area.
3. Reduction in deaths of adolescents & young adults.	Reduce to 16.8 per 100,000 for 10–14 yr olds; 43.2 per 100,000 for 15–19 yr olds; 57.3 per 100,000 for 20–24 yr olds.	No data	?	Identify common causes of death among adolescents & young adults in the target area.
4. Reduce maternal deaths.	Reduce to 3.3 per 100,000.	No data	?	Identify common causes of maternal morbidity in the target area.

				Develop a regional health and wellness center, affiliated with area hospitals, to provide prenatal care pregnant women who are underserved.
5. Reduction in maternal illness & complications due to pregnancy.	Reduce.	No data	?	Identify common causes of maternal illness & pregnancy complications in the target area. Develop a regional health and wellness center, affiliated with area hospitals, to provide prenatal care to pregnant women who are underserved.
6. Increase the proportion of pregnant women who receive early & adequate prenatal care.	Increase to 90% in first trimester; and 90% overall.	In 1998, prenatal care in the first trimester was received by 71.5% in Lake County, 71.2% in LaPorte County, & 76.3% in Porter County (Indiana Natality, 2000).	X	Develop a regional health and wellness center, affiliated with area hospitals, to provide prenatal care to pregnant women who are underserved. Educate middle and high school students regarding increased pregnancy outcomes associated with early prenatal care.
7. Increase the proportion of pregnant women who attend a series of prepared childbirth classes.	Increase.	No data	?	Provide childbirth class information with prenatal care. Offer childbirth classes at health clinic site.
8. Increase the proportion of very low birth weight	Increase to 90%.	In 1998, the proportion of VLBW (<1500 gms) was slightly more		Develop a regional health and wellness center, affiliated with area hos-

continues

TABLE 5-3 Needs Assessment: Maternal, Child, and Family Health and Wellness *continued*

HP 2010 OBJECTIVES	TARGET	DATA ASSESSED	NEED	RECOMMENDATIONS
(VLBW) infants born at level III hospitals or subspecialty perinatal centers.		than 1% in Indiana. 3.0% of infants born to Black women & 1.2% of infants born to White women were classified as VLBW (Indiana Natality, 2000).		pitals, to provide prenatal care to pregnant women who are underserved. Encourage legislators to institute PRAMS in Indiana.
9. Reduce cesarean births among low risk (full-term, singleton, vertex presentation) women.	Decrease to 15.5%.	No data	?	Offer information regarding labor & childbirth at prenatal visits so pregnant women will be able to anticipate labor & delivery realistically. Encourage regular prenatal visits to observe early for development of complications of pregnancy.
10. Reduce low birth weight & very low birth weight.	Reduce low birth weight to 5.0% & very low birth weight to 0.9%.	In Lake County LBW infant births were 8.7%.(Health Resources, 2000).In Gary 10.8% were LBW & 2.4% were VLBW (Indiana Natality, 2000).	X	Develop a regional health and wellness center, affiliated with area hospitals, to provide prenatal care to pregnant women who are underserved. Encourage regular prenatal visits to observe early for development of complications of pregnancy.
11. Reduce preterm births.	Reduce to 7.6%.	1998 preterm births were Lake County 9.0%; LaPorte County 5.7%; Porter County 6.3% (Indiana Natality, 2000).	?	Develop a regional health and wellness center, affiliated with area hospitals, to provide prenatal care to pregnant women who are underserved.

Objective	Target			Strategies
12. Increase the proportion of mothers who achieve a recommended weight gain during their pregnancies.	Increase.	No data	?	Encourage regular prenatal visits to observe early for development of complications of pregnancy. Offer pregnant women admission into drug rehab programs as illicit drug use contributes to preterm birth & childbirth complications. Develop a regional health and wellness center, affiliated with area hospitals, to provide prenatal care to pregnant women who are underserved. Make available access to food banks and programs such as WIC to assist pregnant women to eat a nutritious diet.
13. Increase the percentage of healthy full-term infants who are put down to sleep on their backs.	Increase to 70%.	No data	?	Educate middle and high school students regarding proper infant sleep and the risk of SIDS. Educate pregnant women at prenatal visits and at well-child visits and immunization clinics regarding infant sleep and the risk of SIDS. Put posters in child care centers and other places infants are cared for to educate both care givers and parents.

continues

TABLE 5-3 Needs Assessment: Maternal, Child, and Family Health and Wellness *continued*

HP 2010 OBJECTIVES	TARGET	DATA ASSESSED	NEED	RECOMMENDATIONS
14. Reduce the occurrence of developmental disabilities.	Reduce.	No data	?	Develop a regional health and wellness center, affiliated with area hospitals, to provide prenatal care to pregnant women who are underserved. Developmental difficulties are associated with preterm births, and illicit drug & alcohol use during pregnancy.
15. Reduce the occurrence of spina bifida & other neural tube defects (NTDs).	Reduce to 3 new cases per 10,000 live births.	No data	?	Make available access to food banks and programs such as WIC to assist pregnant women to eat a nutritious diet. Educate middle and high school students regarding proper nutrition prior to conception & during pregnancy, especially sources of folic acid.
16. Increase the proportion of pregnancies begun with an optimum folic acid level.	Increase to 80%.	No data	?	Educate middle and high school students regarding proper nutrition prior to conception & during pregnancy, especially sources of folic acid. Educate young women who seek health care health regarding proper

17. Increase abstinence from alcohol, cigarettes & illicit drugs among pregnant women.	Increase to 90%.	1998 Alcohol use during pregnancy by county: Lake 0.9%, LaPorte 0.8%, Porter 0.6%. Smoking during pregnancy by county: Lake 17.3%, LaPorte 26.33%, Porter 26.33% (Indiana Natality, 2000).	?	nutrition prior to conception & during pregnancy, especially sources of folic acid. Increase availability of programs to assist women who have drug &/or alcohol dependency. Provide information about these programs in clinics that provide prenatal care.
18. Reduce the occurrence of fetal alcohol syndrome (FAS).		1998 Alcohol use during pregnancy by county: Lake 0.9%, LaPorte 0.8%, Porter 0.6% (Indiana Natality, 2000). No data on incidence of FAS.	?	Participation in PRAMS.
19. Increase the proportion of women who breast-feed their babies.	Increase to 75%.	In 1998 in Indian a 55.9% of all mothers were breast feeding when discharged from the hospital. Of these 58% were White & 36.6% were Black (Indiana Natality, 2000).	X	
20. Ensure appropriate newborn bloodspot screening, follow-up testing, & referral to services.		No data	?	

continues

TABLE 5-3 Needs Assessment: Maternal, Child, and Family Health and Wellness *continued*

HP 2010 OBJECTIVES	TARGET	DATA ASSESSED	NEED	RECOMMENDATIONS
21. Reduce hospitalization for life-threatening sepsis among children age 4 yrs & under with sickling hemoglobinopathies.	Reduce occurrence.	No data	?	
22. Increase the proportion of children with special health care needs who have access to a medical home.	Increase proportion.	Indiana does not currently belong to the Pregnancy Risk Assessment Monitoring System (PRAMS). PRAMS would provide data to be used to improve the health of mothers & infants in reducing adverse birth outcomes (Center for Disease Control, Reproductive Health, 2000).	?	Participation in PRAMS would provide needed data.
23. Increase the proportion of territories & states that have service systems for children with special health care needs.	Increase to 100%.	Indiana does not currently belong to the Pregnancy Risk Assessment Monitoring System (PRAMS). In Indiana availability of developmental therapies after 3 yrs of age are subject to state funding which is not guaranteed (Nardi, et al, 2001).	?	Participation in PRAMS would provide needed data.

After studying the chart, more data may be sought for those areas for which the team was unable to find statistics. In this example, there are 13 target benchmarks lacking data. If all available secondary data sources have been utilized and the data is still unknown, the team must choose between collecting the data firsthand themselves or eliminating those benchmarks where they cannot identify needs. By eliminating those with missing benchmarks, the chart is reduced to a smaller size that reflects only the areas with known data. In the case of the data here, the chart would be reduced from 23 benchmarks to 10. The team may then focus energy on those with known data and determine exact areas where the health and well-being of women, infants, and children exist in the community of reference. In this way, the list of 23 benchmarks is reduced to four known areas of need. Certainly this poses the risk of forgetting to address the missing data and may not be in the best interests of the population being assessed. This choice rests with the assessment team. The following excerpt from the assessment team's report illustrates how the comparison of data to *Healthy People 2010* benchmarks can be used to identify community strengths, areas of concern, and priority needs concerning maternal child and family health and wellness:

> Working poor families in the county account for only 1% of recipients of family planning services. Family planning services by clinics and county health departments are limited and scarce. The state ranks low among the states in degree of decrease in teen pregnancy rates. Contraceptive devices are not covered by almost one-fourth of health care polices in the state. Although almost half of high school students have had sexual intercourse at least once, almost half of sexually active teens do not regularly use a condom at intercourse.
>
> Percentage of low birth weight newborns remains a problem; at 8.7% in the county, it is higher than the Healthy People target of 5.0%. Percentage of premature births is also higher than Healthy People 2010 targets. Almost 40% of mothers in the city did not receive prenatal care in the first trimester; approximately 24% of mothers in another county and 20% of mothers in the third county did not receive prenatal care in the first trimester. Over 17% of pregnant women smoked during their pregnancy. Most mothers in the state do not breast feed by discharge from the hospital. The infant mortality rate for Black infants is higher than the national rate of 10.3, and higher than the mortality rate for White infants. Most telling, the state does not belong to the Pregnancy Risk Assessment Monitoring System (PRAMS), which provides data that State Health Departments can use to improve pregnancy outcomes for both women and children."
> (Nardi et al., 2001, pp. 74–75)

This chapter applies the steps of the Ontario Needs Impact Based Model to the assessment of women's, children's, and families' health and well-being needs. The health and well-being of children is assessed within the overall context of family functioning, including pregnancy planning, responsible sexual behaviors, maternal care, and family health.

KEY POINTS

◆ Social, physical, and environmental domains of maternal, child, and family health and wellness must be included in any assessment of the community health needs of the child-bearing family.

◆ Social factors that impact maternal, child, and family health and wellness include parenting style and caregiving, social support, SES level and marital status of the child-bearing family, sexual activity, and lifestyle choices, such as maternal smoking, drug, and alcohol use during pregnancy.

◆ Physical factors that impact maternal, child, and family health and wellness include proper prenatal care and maternal nutrition, breastfeeding practices, prenatal drug and alcohol exposure, and chronic illnesses and disabilities of children.

◆ Environmental factors that impact maternal, child, and family health and wellness include neighborhood and community violence, access to quality schools, and employment opportunities for the parents.

◆ When identifying the need for a health assessment, the assessment team must decide what part of the family unit will be included, as this will determine not only the *Healthy People 2010* goals chosen as benchmarks, but which data is collected and which sources are used.

◆ Specific *Healthy People 2010* goals to be used to assess maternal, child, and family health and wellness include goals 9, 13, 14, 16, 17, and 25. Goals 7 and 15 also contain objectives that can be used to guide the assessment of the quality of life in the neighborhoods.

◆ In determining the purpose of the maternal, child, and family health assessment, the team must also choose a target population, such as pregnant and parenting women between the ages of 15 and 25, or infants and toddlers, or low-income families.

◆ The health and well-being of children should be assessed within the overall context of family functioning, including pregnancy planning, responsible sexual behaviors, maternal care and family health, and safe neighborhoods.

REFERENCES

Adler, N. E., Boyce, T., Chesney, M. A., Cohen, S., Folkman, S., Kahn, R. L., & Syme, S. L. (1994). Socioeconomic status and health: The challenge of the gradient. *American Psychologist, 49*, 15–24.

American Academy of Pediatrics. (1999). *The medical home and early intervention: Linking services for children with special needs.* Elk Grove Village, IL: AAP, 1999.

American Academy of Pediatrics Committee on Substance Abuse. (1995). Drug-exposed infants. *Pediatrics, 96*, 364–367.

Beaudry, M., Dufour, R., & Marcoux, S. (1995). Relation between infant feeding and infections during the first 6 months of life. *Journal of Pediatrics, 126*, 191–197.

Boyd-Franklin, N. (1987). Group therapy for black women: A therapeutic support model. *American Journal of Orthopsychiatry, 57*, 394–401.

Boyle, M., & Zola, G. (1996). *Personal nutrition* (3rd ed.). Minneapolis, MN: West.

Bronfenbrenner, U. (1979). Contexts of childrearing. *American Psychologist, 34*, 844–850.

Bronfenbrenner, U. (1990). *Who cares for children?* (Annual Report). Sapporo, Japan: Faculty of education, Hokkaido University.

Brown, S., & Eisenberg, L. (Eds.). (1995). The best intentions: Unintended pregnancy and the well being of children and families. Washington, DC: National Academy Press.

Brunham, R., Holmes, K., & Embree, J. (1990). Sexually transmitted diseases in pregnancy. In K. Holmes, P. Mardh, & Sparling, P. (Eds.), *Sexually transmitted disease* (2nd ed., pp. 771–801). New York: McGraw-Hill.

Camas, O., Cheung, L., & Lieberman, E. (1995). The role of lifestyle in preventing low birth weight. *Future Child, 5*, 121–138.

Centers for Disease Control and Prevention. (1995). Health insurance coverage and receipt of preventative health services—United States, 1993. *Morbidity and Mortality Weekly Report, 44*, 219–225.

Centers for Disease Control and Prevention, Reproductive Health Information Source. (2000). *Pregnancy risk assessment monitoring system* [online]. Available: http://www.cdc.gov/nccdphp/drh/srv_prams.htm.

Dawson, D. (1991). Family structure and children's health and wellbeing: Data from 1988. National Health Interview Survey on Child Health. *Journal of Marriage and the Family, 53*, 573–584.

Department of Education. (1991). *Preparing young children for success: Guideposts for achieving our first national goal. An America 2000 Education Strategy.*

Washington, DC: Office of Planning, Budget and Education—Office of Educational Research and Improvement (ED):

Dewey, K., Heinig, M., & Nommsen, L. (1993). Maternal weight-loss patterns during prolonged lactation. *American Journal of Clinical Nutrition, 58,* 162–166.

Donovan, E., & Sanders, B. (1999). Marital status and health outcomes 1997–1998. *Children and Family Health Services Maternal and Child Health Report, 4,* 1–3.

Feldman, R., Teclaw, R., & Gamache, R. (2000). *Indiana natality report.* Indianapolis: Indiana State Department of Health.

Fiese, B., & Sameroff, J. (1989). Family context in pediatric psychology: A transactional perspective. *Journal of Pediatric Psychology, 14,* 293–314.

Foege, W. H., Rosenberg, M. L., & Mercy, J. A. (1995). Public health and violence prevention. *Current Issues in Public Health, 1,* 2–9.

Garbarino, J. (1990). The human ecology of early risk. In S. Meisels & J. Shonkoff (Eds.), *Handbook of early childhood intervention* (pp. 78–96). Cambridge: Cambridge University Press.

Garbarino, J. and Associates. (1992). *Children and families in the social environment* (2nd ed.). New York: Aldine-deGruyter.

Goldenberg, R., Andrews, W., Yuan, A. & MacKay, H. (1997). Sexually transmitted diseases and adverse outcomes of pregnancy. *Clinics in Perinatology: Infections in Perinatology, 24,* 23–41.

Gottman, J., & Katz, L. (1989). Effects of marital discord on young children's peer interruption and health. *Developmental Psychology, 25,* 373–381.

Grad, R., & Hill, I. (1992). Financing maternal and child health care in the United States, In C. Blakely, S. Brown, & J. Kotch (Eds.), *A pound of prevention: The case for universal maternity care in the U.S.* Washington, DC: American Public Health Association.

Hamburg, M. (1998). Eliminating racial and ethnic disparities in health: Response to the Presidential Initiative on Race. *Public Health Reports, 113,* 372–375.

Harkey, A. (1997). Pregnant and HIV-positive: A case study. *Journal of Maternal Child Nursing, 2* (22), 85–88.

Health Resources and Services Administration. (2000). *Community health status report: Lake County Indiana July 2000.* Merrifield, VA: U.S. Department of Health and Human Services.

HHS, Administration on Children, Youth, and Families. Child Maltreatment. (1994). *Reports from the states to the National Child Abuse and Neglect Data System (1997).* Washington, DC: U.S. Government Printing Office.

Hoyert, D. (1996). Medical and life-style risk factors affecting fetal mortality, 1989–90. Vital and health statistics 20 data. *National Vital Statistics System, 31,* 1–32.

Indiana Natality Report. (2000). Indianapolis: Indiana State Dept. of Health.

Jones, K. (1986). Fetal alcohol syndrome. *Pediatric Review, 8,* 122–126.

Kent-Wilkerson, A. (1996). Spousal abuse/homicide. A current issues in health risk management. *Journal of Psychosocial Nursing, 34,* 12–15.

Kochanek, K., Maurer, J., & Rosenberg, H. (1994). Why did Black life expectancy decline from 1984 through 1989 in the United States? *American Journal of Public Health, 84,* 938–944.

Kost, K., Landry, D., & Darroch, J. (1998). Predicting maternal behaviors during pregnancy: Does intention matter? *Family Planning Perspectives, 30,* 79–88.

Lundsberg, L., Bracken, M., & Saftlas, A. (1997). Low-to-moderate gestational alcohol use and intrauterine growth retardation, low birth weight and preterm delivery. *Annals of Epidemiology, 7,* 498–508.

Miller, F. (1988). Network structure support: Its relationship to the psychosocial development of black females. *Journal of Applied Social Psychology, 15,* 448–465.

Montgomery, D., & Splett, P. (1997). Economic benefits of breast-feeding infants enrolled in WIC. *Journal of the American Dietetic Association, 97,* 379–385.

Mothers' Survey. (1998). Ross Products Division, Abbott Laboratory, Inc.

Nardi, D., Sutherland, T., Tippy, F., Strupeck, D., et al. (2001). *Needs assessment of the health and well being of the Northwest Indiana region.* Indiana University Northwest Shared Vision Research and Service Task Forces. Unpublished manuscript.

Nath, P., Whitman, T., Borkowski, J., & Schellenbach, C. (1990). *Understanding adolescent parenting; the dimension and functions of social support.* Unpublished manuscript, University of Notre Dame, Indiana.

National Education Goals Panel. (1999). *The National Education Goals Report: Building a Nation of Learners.* Washington, DC: National Education Goals Panel.

National Heart, Lung and Blood Institute. (1995). *Chronic obstructive lung disease.* Washington, DC: National Institutes for Health (NIH Publication no. 95-2020).

National Rural Health Association (NRHA). (1998). *Bringing resources to bear on the changing care system: Conference proceedings from 2nd annual rural minority health conference.* Kansas City, MO: NRHA.

Nelson, M. (1994). Economic impoverishment as a health risk: Methodologic and conceptual issues. *Advances in Nursing Science, 16,* 1–12.

Palfrey, J. (1995). *Community child health.* Westpoint, CT: Praeger.

Pearson, J. (1986). The definition and measurement of social support. *Journal of Counseling and Development, 64,* 390–395.

Riegel, K. (1975). Toward a dialectical theory of development. *Human Development, 18,* 50–64.

Reinhardt, U. (1994). Coverage and access in health care reform. *New England Journal of Medicine, 330,* 1452–1453.

Riley, R., & Shalala, D. (1994). *Joint statement on school health.* Washington, DC: U.S. Department of Education and Health and Human Services.

Ruppert, E. (1997). Early intervention. In H. Wallace, R. Biehl, J. MacQueen, & J. Blackman (Eds.), *Children with disabilities and chronic illness* (pp. 338–345). St. Louis, MO: Mosby.

Sameroff, J., & Fiese, B. (1990). Transactional regulation and early intervention. In S. Meisels & J. Shonkoff (Eds.), *Handbook of early childhood intervention* (pp. 119–149). Cambridge: Cambridge University Press.

Schorr, L. (1989). *Within our reach: Breaking the cycle of disadvantage.* New York: Doubleday.

Singh, G., Kochanek, K., & MacDorman, M. (1996). Advance report of final mortality statistics, 1994. *Monthly Vital Statistics Report, 45 (3S).* Hyattsville, MD: National Center for Health Statistics.

Stock, J., Bell, M., Boyer, D., & Connell, F. (1997). Adolescent pregnancy and sexual risk-taking among sexually abused girls. *Family Planning Perspectives, 29,* 1–11.

Stratton, K., Howe, C., & Battaglia, F. (Eds.). (1996). *Fetal alcohol syndrome: Diagnosis, epidemiology, prevention and treatment.* Washington, DC: National Academy Press.

Unger, D., & Wasserman, L. (1988). The relation of family and partner support to the adjustment of adolescent mothers. *Child Development, 59,* 1056–1060.

U.S. Census Bureau (2000). *Lake County quick facts from the US Census Bureau* [online]. Available: http://quickfacts.census.gov/qfd/states/18/18089.html.

U.S. Department of Health and Human Services (2000). *Healthy People 2010.* Washington, DC: U.S. Government Printing Office.

U.S. General Accounting Office (1998). *Health insurance coverage leads to increased health care access to children.* GAO/HEHS-98-14. Washington, DC: General Accounting Office.

Ventura, S., Martin, J., Curtin, S., & Mathews, T. (1999). Births: Final data for 1997. *National Vital Statistics Reports, 45* (18).

Wallace, H., & Gittler, J. (1998). Federal legislation for children with special health care needs and their families: Past, present, and future. In H. Wallace, R. Biehl, J. MacQueen, & J. Blackman (Eds.), *Children with disabilities and chronic illness.* St. Louis, MO: Mosby.

Wisconsin Association for Perinatal Care (WAPC). (2000). *Positions statement: Preconceptual care.* Madison: Wisconsin Association for Perinatal Care.

World Health Assembly (1996). *Prevention of violence: Public health priority.* Forty-Ninth World Health Assembly, Geneva.

Zuckerman, B. (1998). Marijuana and cigarette smoking during pregnancy: Neonatal effects. In I. Chasnoff, (Ed.), *Drugs, alcohol, pregnancy, and parenting.* Boston: Kluwer Academic Publishers.

Chapter

6

ASSESSING COMMUNITY
HEALTH AND WELLNESS

Daniel Lowery

 LEARNING OBJECTIVES

At the conclusion of this chapter, the reader will be able to:

◆ Locate the community-based indicators movement within the contexts of four larger societal trends.

◆ Describe steps that are required in developing community-based
indicators.

◆ Understand alternatives that are suggested by certain exemplary
sets of community-based indicators.

◆ Critique alternative sets of community-based indicators.

KEY TERMS

Carrying capacity	Outcomes
Community intervention	Quality of life
Community status reports	Service learning
Continuous improvement	Sponsor
Dashboard indicators	Steering committee
Health community	Strong democracy
Healthy People	Sustainability
Indicators	Sustainable development

F our societal trends are examined in this chapter. Each has contributed to the growing use of community-based indicators. Further, 11 questions that communities typically face in developing indicators are posed. Several initiatives are described in some detail in the course of examining these questions. Exemplary sets of indicator categories are also illustrated, and the indicators that pertain specifically to health in each of these examples are presented. As we shall see, a number of alternatives with respect to approach, theory, design, and use are available to decision makers who elect to pursue initiatives of this kind. Care should be exercised in choosing among these several alternatives, however. The best indicators are those that are tailored to the needs of the subject community.

THE COMMUNITY-BASED INDICATORS MOVEMENT

By one estimation, over 200 communities in the United States have developed community-based **indicators** (i.e., measures that reflect the condition of a system) of one type or another (Oregon Progress Board, 1999, p. 1; Besleme & Mullin, 1997). The first national conference on the subject took place in Denver in 1996 and attracted participants from 150 different communities (Strong, 1997, p. 19). This development can be attributed, in part, to the federal government's *Healthy People* initiative. However, larger societal trends have prompted the development of community-based indicators as well. In fact, four tendencies over the past 30 years have contributed to the kinds of data gathering, assessment, and community-based action that are promoted in the *Healthy People* initiative and other related endeavors.

The first of these trends pertains to our collective understanding of the concept of human flourishing, which has expanded greatly over time. This is evident, for instance, in our changing conception of human rights. Internationally, the Nuremberg War Crimes Trials and the Helsinki Declaration on Human Rights have codified the view that some human rights are, in fact, inalienable. In this country, debates pertaining to the extent to which housing, employment, and health care represent constitutionally protected rights have attained status on the public policy agenda at various times over the course of the past 50 years. Even some contract theorists now point to a broad set of needs that extends well beyond the political rights that are embodied in the Constitution. David Held, for instance, defines "nautonomy" as "the asymmetrical production and distribution of life-chances which limit and erode the possibilities of political participation" (1995, p. 171). In contrast, autonomy is embodied in certain "empowering rights" or "entitlement capacities." Further, the "good" is reflected in the distribution and achievement of individual life-chances (p. 223). Held goes on to argue that the experiences of autonomy and nautonomy take place in six distinct spheres of an individual's life: the body; social welfare; culture or cultural life; civic associations; the economy; and the organization of violence and coercive relations (pp. 176–183). He thus extends the idea of the social contract beyond the narrow domain of the political. And in doing so, he cites categories that are reflected, in one way or another, in many community-based indicators or **community status** reports.

This expanded conception of human flourishing is also reflected in a growing disillusionment with money as the primary or sole measure of human happiness. National and international metrics, such as gross national product and gross domestic product, are no longer viewed as sufficient (Besleme & Mullin, 1997). As is noted in the introduction to the Northwest Indiana Quality of Life Council's indicators report, "'Quality of life' is ultimately more important than 'standard of living.' 'Standard of living' refers solely to the private domain and to the disposable income that we use to purchase things individually. 'Quality of life' refers to the public domain. It's the sum of things that people purchase collectively, such as the health-care system and those things we need to live but do not purchase, like the air we breathe" (Northwest Indiana Quality of Life Council, 2000, p. 6). The popular management literature points to a similar disenchantment with financial measures of well-being at the level of the individual (Covey, 1989; Block, 1987; Handy, 1998; Moore, 1992). In and of itself, money is no longer believed by many to be reflective of well-being, thus the need for more comprehensive sets of community-based indicators.

The systematic focus of many indicators initiatives is also reflective of an appreciation for the interconnectedness of the many factors that together contribute to a high quality of life. First attaining prominence in the 1960s, systems theory rejects the closed metaphor of the machine. It holds that social and environmental systems are more like living organisms. They are affected by a broad range of factors and interact with these factors in complex ways (Kast & Rosenzweig, 1972; Katz & Kahn, 1966).

Systems theory lies at the heart of the concept of sustainability, which, as we shall see, undergirds many community-based indicators initiatives. A systems model is used to illustrate the relationships that exist among the six broad categories that are included in the United Way of America's State of Giving Index. Figure 6-1 is designed to visually capture the dynamic interplay of the (index's 32) indicators.

While the issues they represent are part of the social and economic tapestry of society, the 32 indicators act as interwoven threads within that social fabric. "When one is tattered or weakened, it may undermine the strength of the whole" (United Way of America, 2000, p. 12). A systems model is also featured in the federal government's *Healthy People* initiative to illustrate the interrelationships that exist among six broad categories: biology; individual behavior; the social environment; the physical environment; policies and interventions; and access to healthcare (U.S. Department of Health and Human Services, 2000, pp. 19–20). "Indeed, the underlying premise of Healthy People 2010 is that the health of the individual is almost inseparable from the health of the larger community and that the health of every community in every state and territory determines the overall health status of the nation" (U.S. Department of Health and Human Services, 2000, p. 3). Systems theory is deeply embedded in each of these approaches to the development of national and community-based indicators.

The devolution of some national programs to the state, regional, and local levels of government has also contributed to a growing interest in community-based indicators. The Nixon administration's New Federalism was followed, in turn, by the Reagan Revolution of the 1980s and the Republican Contract with America in the 1990s. Although these developments have been dismissed by some as an abandonment of certain national commitments, others have described them as milestones in the rebirth of a concern for local community. It is in this sense that Benjamin Barber defines **strong democracy** as "politics in the participatory mode, where conflict is resolved in the absence of an independent ground through a participatory process of ongoing, proximate self-legislation, and the creation of a political community capable of transforming dependent, private individuals into free citizens, and partial and private interests into public goods" (1984, p. 132). Strong democracy favors direct

Figure 6-1 ▪ United Way of America State of Giving Index
(United Way of America, 2000, p. 12)

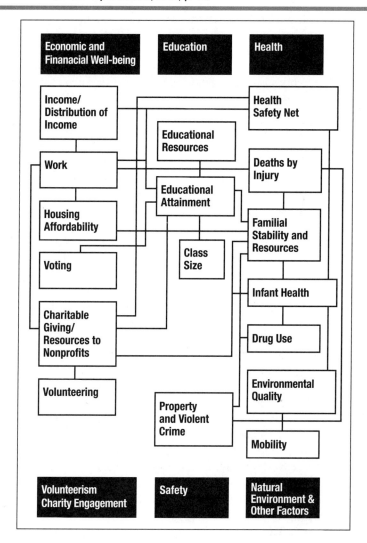

participation over indirect representation in government. It expresses a positive understanding of freedom. It also endorses a broad scope of action for government and the nonprofit community. In Barber's view, our political life can find its fullest expression at the local or community level. He argues that our political concerns should be broad-based, extending well beyond the narrow focus on taxes and spending that has eviscerated our understanding of citizenship. Like other social critics, Barber believes that the citizen is too often conceptualized as little more than a taxpayer or consumer. Consistent with Barber's view, the development and use of indicators in problem-solving activities is reflective of a more complete understanding of one's place in the life of his her local community.

The total quality movement is also consistent with the development of community-based indicators. W. Edwards Deming (1986) and Joseph Juran (1974), who, along with others, contributed so much to the reengineering of business and manufacturing practices in the United States in the 1980s and 1990s, argued that measurement is central to the concept of continuous improvement. "You cannot improve what you do not measure." In the same way that advertising cannot ensure a good product or service, community-based measures that focus solely on the kinds of data that might attract new residents, consumers, and investors to a community cannot alone engender positive change. A community must gather data across a broad front. Further, it is not enough just to gather data; measures of performance must be linked to an improvement planning process. Referring to manufacturing processes, Deming noted that "figures on productivity do not help to improve productivity. . . . [They] are like statistics on accidents. They tell you all about the number of accidents in the home, on the road, and at the work place, but they do not tell you how to reduce the frequency of accidents" (1982, p. 15). Exemplary community-based initiatives include processes that link the gathering of data to action steps of one kind or another.

This new sophistication in the design of performance measures is also reflected in the use of **outcomes** measures in program evaluations. Like other funders, United Way of America is now promoting the articulation of three levels of outcomes by its 44,000 member agencies (Lowery, 2001). In the United Way scheme, "immediate" outcomes are defined as cognitive or affective change; "intermediate" outcomes are defined as behavioral change; and "long-term" outcomes are defined as improved life chances or improved "quality of life." Together, these three levels of outcomes are distinguished from the kinds of output measures on which the nonprofit community has typically relied (i.e., units of service, conformance to specifications, satisfaction, and timeliness) (United Way of America, 1996). The best sets of community-based indicators include measures of cognitive and affective change, behavioral change, and the extent to which the life chances of individuals have been improved and the community's quality of life has been enhanced.

For each of these several reasons, the community-based indicators movement should not be viewed as something that is separate from other developments. It testifies to a more sophisticated understanding of human flourishing. It also reflects a growing appreciation for the interconnectedness of the many factors that contribute to a high quality of life. Further, the community-based indicators movement represents a positive reaction to the ongoing devolution of some federal programs. Finally, it is consistent with an emphasis in the contemporary quality movement on measurement and continuous improvement.

This conceptual location of the community-based indicators movement suggests that it is much more than a passing fad. It may, in fact, be the key to achieving what Benjamin Barber calls strong democracy. More specifically, McKiernan and Plantz contend that community-based indicators can "create unity, ignite commitment from diverse community stakeholders, and lay a solid foundation for future action" (1999). Using similar language, Besleme and Mullin argue that indicators projects can "cultivate a sense of shared responsibility for community health and wellbeing. . . . They (can) help bridge the gap between government and citizens, build important coalitions within communities, (and) draw attention to problems and negative trends before they become damaging" (1997).

DEVELOPING AND USING COMMUNITY-BASED INDICATORS

There is more than one way to develop and use community-based indicators. In fact, the best sets of indicators are those that are tailored to the needs of the communities to which they speak. Community-based indicators will be useful only if they are meaningful. They must be situated in time and place; context makes a difference. This is not to say that anything goes, however. Drawing on the experience of *Healthy People* initiatives, the U.S. Department of Health and Human Services coined the acronym MAP-IT to delineate key steps in the development and use of community-based indicators. Participants must **M**obilize individuals and organizations who care about the health of their community into a coalition; **A**ssess the areas of greatest need; **P**lan a vision, an approach, a strategy, and action steps; **I**mplement a plan; and **T**rack progress over time (Office of Disease Prevention and Health Promotion, 2001, p. 6). In the same vein, we now have enough experience with indicators to identify 11 questions that organizers of community-based initiatives should be prepared to answer.

1. Who will sponsor the development of the indicators?

2. How will the project be funded?

3. Who will guide the development of the indicators?

4. What theory will guide their development?

5. How will "community" be defined?

6. What categories of measurement will be adopted?

7. What kinds of indicators will be selected?

8. What kinds of comparisons will be made?

9. What kinds of background information will accompany the data?

10. How will the indicators be used?

11. How will the indicators be maintained?

Each of these questions will be addressed in turn. Several exemplary sets of indicator categories will be described in detail as well. Health-related indicators will also be broken out for closer examination.

WHO WILL SPONSOR THE DEVELOPMENT OF THE INDICATORS?

Sponsors serve two vital functions: (1) they host the initial meeting or set of meetings; (2) they marshal the resources that will be needed to support the initiative through its preliminary stages of development.

With respect to the first function, the sponsor must have sufficient standing in the community to secure the cooperation of key decision makers. Some Health Departments have played this role. For instance, the Pasadena, California Public Health Department issued invitations to a summit that drew over 150 citizens representing various neighborhoods and a diverse group of interests (Besleme & Mullin, 1997). The nonprofit community can perform this function as well. In Marathon County, Wisconsin, the United Way affiliate assumed the lead in organizing an indicators initiative (Community Planning Council of Marathon County, 1999). In Vermont, the state government led the way with the assistance of the Annie E. Casey Foundation (Hogan, 1999, p. 1). The metropolitan planning organizations of Northwest Indiana and Reno, Nevada (Besleme & Mullin, 1997), both recognized a need for regional problem-solving initiatives; they organized meetings that led to the eventual development of indicators. Representatives of the business community can also serve as sponsors. In Jacksonville, Florida, the chamber of commerce called for a planning meeting and raised funds for an indicators project (Besleme & Mullin, 1997). Clearly, many different kinds of organizations can serve as sponsors. Only rarely, however, do initiatives begin at the grassroots level or with organizations that stand at the margins of community life. More often than not, established organizations with standing in their respective communities play this role.

A sponsor must also be able to secure funds to support an initial round of meetings. This can often be accomplished within the context of the sponsor's mission, thereby providing a rationale for the allocation of agency or organization funds. This is true in the case of public Health Departments, some nonprofit organizations, metropolitan planning organizations, and chambers of commerce and other business-related organizations. In other cases, a sponsor may need to secure a planning grant from a unit of government or a foundation. In this role, a sponsor can sometimes provide grant writing services or serve as the project's fiscal agent. In Pasadena, the Health Department drew on resources provided by the California Healthy Cities Project (Strong, 1995, p. 19). In Northwest Indiana, the Northwestern Indiana Regional Planning Commission secured a planning grant from Region V of the Environmental Protection Agency.

Although a sponsor is often required to play a critical role early in the development of an initiative, its preeminent position need not be long-lived. A new entity is often established to oversee the project's development. This was true in Pasadena, where a coalition eventually developed a quality of life index for the city, a planning matrix, and a communications plan. In Madison County, Wisconsin, the United Way effort led to the formation of a loose-knit coalition that included representatives from local government, the business community, several health care organizations, and a community foundation. The chamber of commerce initiative in Jacksonville, Florida, led to the creation of the Jacksonville Community Council, which went on to develop a comprehensive set of 74 indicators (Besleme & Mullin, 1997). In Northwest Indiana, a series of community meetings led to the formation of a nonprofit organization called the Quality of Life Council, which is now chaired on a rotating basis by the presidents and chancellors of the region's six colleges and universities. The same approach was adopted in Reno, Nevada, where the Truckee Meadows Regional Planning Commission handed the initiative over to Truckee Meadows Tomorrow, a nonprofit coalition of some 50 clubs and organizations (Besleme & Mullin, 1997). Although short-lived, the sponsor's contribution in each of these cases proved critical to its eventual success.

How Will the Project Be Funded?

Although a sponsor's financial contribution may be sufficient to host an initial series of planning meetings, additional funds will be needed to fully develop and implement a community-based indicators initiative. Through publication, the Marathon County project cost $33,000. Another $13,400 was subsequently raised to promote the initiative (Community

Planning Council of Marathon County, 1999, p. 1). The indicators project in Northwest Indiana cost $20,000. The funds needed to support an initiative can vary, however, based on several factors, including the number of indicators selected, the kinds of data that will be gathered, the expertise of staff and consultants, and the publication strategy that is adopted. Because these kinds of expenses can be anticipated, however, they can be factored into the development of a financial plan. Each will be addressed in turn.

Due to a lack of funds, most initiatives rely on public sources of data. Tax dollars are used to gather and maintain public databases. As fiscal pressures grow, however, the resources needed to develop and maintain high-quality data at the federal, state, and local levels of government can come under pressure (Strong, 1997). Protecting these resources requires that political leaders understand the contribution that good data can make to sound decision making and the effect, in turn, that sound decision making can have on the need for public funding over time. For example, the connection between smoking cessation programs, which often draw on public resources, and Medicaid and Medicare expenditures must be made explicit. Similarly, the long-term effects of combined sewer systems, water quality, and the costs of remediation must be made clear. A great deal of information that is maintained by federal, state, regional, and local units of government is available at little or no cost. In some cases, however, planning teams may decide that supplemental data of a specific or local nature is required. For instance, there may be an interest in local attitudes pertaining to racial diversity, social justice, or satisfaction with public services, data that is not gathered on a routine basis. Consequently, the steering committee may need to contract for the design of a survey instrument or the administration of a telephone or in-person survey. It may be possible to secure a foundation grant or a contribution from a local business for this purpose. Alternatively, the steering committee can approach a local college or university with a request that a survey be designed and administered as part of a **service learning** or community service project. Service learning refers to "a method of teaching through which students apply newly acquired academic skills and knowledge to address real-life needs in their own communities" (Payne, 2000, pp. 3–4).

Staff support may also be needed. In the Marathon County initiative, a research analyst was hired on a temporary basis to provide staff support to the steering committee that guided the overall effort (Community Planning Council of Marathon County, 1999). The Northwest Indiana initiative contracted for the services of a local research institute that is associated with the Roman Catholic Diocese of Gary. When its grant from the

Environmental Protection Agency was exhausted, the Northwest Indiana Quality of Life Council secured a series of smaller grants from local and national foundations and the Indiana Association of United Ways. These funds were supplemented by contributions from several large industries located in the region.

These same sources of funds can be used to finance the publication of indicators reports. It is axiomatic that high-quality reports, which include such features as a card stock base, graphs, charts, pictures, multiple fonts, and several colors, invite media attention, wide distribution, prominent display, and use. These kinds of reports are also costly. Mailing costs must be calculated into the overall cost of publication as well. Electronic publishing represents, at best, a low-cost complement to hard copy distribution. Whereas the initial publication of a hard copy report is often orchestrated to attract the attention of the media and key decision makers, the electronic version of an indicators report will best serve as resource material for a broader range of users.

Adequate funding is essential to the success of an indicators initiative. Each of the above categories of cost needs to be accounted for if an indicators project is to be successful. Preparing grant proposals and soliciting funds can be a time-consuming, difficult, and, sometimes, thankless task, however. Indeed, the lack of stable sources of funds may represent the Achilles heel of the indicators movement. Reliable funding sources are needed to gather, analyze, and publish data. Susan Strong of the Center for Economic Conversion has proposed that federal block grants be used for this purpose (1995). It may also be possible to craft certain mandates into existing laws, regulations, and grants to produce the same result. For instance, the promotion of a broad-based community planning initiative could be incorporated into the requirements of some health, environmental, transportation, and public safety programs. The potential value of this strategy is reflected in the King County Benchmarks initiative. In 1991, the State of Washington directed King County and its 35 cities and towns to develop a 20-year plan for growth. Individual communities were then required to develop plans consistent with the county's vision. A Benchmark Committee was formed, which included representatives from the business community, the nonprofit sector, and various citizens groups. It eventually developed 45 indicators pertaining to land use, affordable housing, economic development, the environment, and transportation (Besleme & Mullin, 1997). If the categorical nature of these various programs could be overcome, well-designed mandates could provide access to funding streams that would be much more reliable than the current mix of public and private funding.

Who Will Guide the Development of the Indicators?

Although a sponsor is needed to issue the call for participation in a community-based initiative and coalitions are essential to sustaining these efforts, a smaller group of individuals is typically asked to select a guiding theory, oversee the project, develop a selection criteria, and choose the indicators with respect to which data will be gathered. Typically, these several tasks are divided between a **steering committee** and support staff.

The steering committee should be broad-based to ensure that the indicator categories and the indicators selected are comprehensive in nature. Indicators that focus too narrowly on environmental concerns, health issues, or the interests of the business community will not serve the larger community as well as a more complete set of indicators. In fact, complementary sets of indicators are needed to tease out the correlations that exist between and among various indicator domains (i.e., health and environmental quality, education and employment, citizen involvement and public safety, etc.)

A lack of credibility will very likely attend to exclusive undertakings of this kind as well. If trust between certain sectors of the community is already strained, a preemptive attempt to define well-being for the community as a whole will very likely be met with indifference or outright hostility. In this vein, it has been suggested that one man's "economic development" is another man's "suburban sprawl." Similarly, housing rehabilitation can be characterized either as "neighborhood development" or "gentrification." Parties representing different perspectives need to be engaged in the development of indicator categories and in the identification of individual indicators if they are to contribute to true problem-solving. For both of these reasons, the steering committee that is formed should be broad-based.

At the same time, the leadership of the steering committee should have sufficient standing in the community to engender confidence in the project and command attention at its completion. In the Northwest Indiana initiative, the chancellor of a local university chaired the steering committee. The committee also included influential members of the business community, representatives of the social services, environmental activists, educators, and local government officials. Working together, these individuals commanded the level of attention that is required if an indicators initiative is to have a positive impact on the life of a community.

In most cases, members of the steering committee do not need to undertake personally the detailed research, data gathering, or analysis that initiatives of this kind require. The steering committee is generally assisted in this work by paid staff or volunteers. This staff support can come in several different forms. It is often secured through university-based research institutes. As noted above, private consultants are sometimes used as well. Staff support can also be provided by a local metropolitan planning organization. Alternatively, the energies of graduate students can be tapped as part of service learning projects associated with various kinds of courses (e.g., statistics, policy analysis, planning, etc.). Finally, the responsibility for developing certain indicator categories can be delegated to existing entities. Thus, a broad-based planning body with an interest in law enforcement could be asked to assume the lead in developing a set of indicators pertaining to public safety. In the same way, a United Way affiliate could take on the responsibility for developing a set of indicators pertaining to family life. And an informal network of health care providers could be asked to develop a set of indicators pertaining to health.

Even when this last option is adopted, however, a steering committee is still needed to perform several key tasks: (1) it adopts the theory that will guide the development of the indicator categories; (2) it selects the indicator categories to be developed; (3) the steering committee ensures that the membership of each partner entity is sufficiently broad-based; (4) it establishes guidelines pertaining to such issues as the time periods to be considered, the number of indicators to be adopted, the level of aggregation to be employed, and the reporting format to be used; (5) it sanctions the involvement of partner entities; (6) the steering committee provides resources in support of their efforts; and (7) it monitors their performance.

The importance of the steering committee cannot be overestimated. Like sponsors, funders, and the broad-based coalitions that typically assume the overall lead in initiatives of this kind, steering committees play a critical role in developing comprehensive sets of community-based indicators. They oversee the design, data gathering, analysis, and reporting that, together, convert a recognized need for community-based indicators into reality. In doing so, steering committees link the catalyzing energies of sponsors, funders, and coalitions to the technical and organizational skills of those who perform the staff functions that contribute to the development of community-based indicators.

What Theory Will Guide the Development of the Indicators?

Although many sets of community-based indicators have much in common, differences do exist. These differences are attributable, in large part, to the theories or principles that undergird their development. In fact, three theories now serve this function: the vision set forth in the *Healthy People* initiative; the concept of sustainability; and the somewhat less well-defined concept of quality of life.

A large number of community-based indicators projects are grounded on the idea of the **healthy community**. According to the U.S. Department of Health and Human Services, a "healthy community embraces the belief that health is more than merely an absence of disease; a healthy community includes those elements that enable people to maintain a high quality of life and productivity" (Office of Disease Prevention and Health Promotion, 2001, p. 1). Perhaps not surprisingly, the healthy community or *Healthy People* model is often adopted when Health Departments serve as project sponsors.

The animating ideas behind the ***Healthy People*** movement are twofold: (1) a belief that health is determined by a broad range of physical, environmental, social, economic, and behavioral factors; and (2) a commitment to the community-based amelioration of disparities in health outcomes (Besleme & Mullin, 1997). These concepts are embodied in a series of reports that have been published by the federal government over the course of the past 20 years. *Healthy People: The Surgeon General's Report on Health Promotion and Disease Prevention* was published in 1979. A companion report, *Promoting Health/Preventing Disease: Objectives for the Nation,* was published in 1980. It identified 226 health objectives to be attained by 1990. A successor document, *Healthy People 2000: National Health Promotion and Disease Prevention,* was published in 1990. The Healthy People Consortium, an alliance of over 600 public, private, and nonprofit entities, was consulted in developing the two overarching goals, the 28 specific focus areas, and the 467 objectives of the *Healthy People 2010* initiative (Office of Disease Prevention and Health Promotion, 2001).

The concept of **sustainability** has served as an organizing principle for other indicators initiatives. Sustainability is defined by the President's Commission on Sustainable Development as "an evolving process that improves the economy, the environment, and society for the benefit of current and future generations" (1996). The International Council for Local Economic Initiatives defines **sustainable development** as a program that can be used to "change the process of economic development so that it can ensure a basic quality of life for all people while protecting ecosystems and community systems that make life possible and worthwhile" (International Council for Local Economic Initiatives, 1996).

The most highly acclaimed set of indicators that is based on the principle of sustainability was developed as part of Seattle's Sustainability City Project. In 1990, a group of concerned citizens developed 20 indicators based on their combined potential to contribute to the city's "long-term cultural, economic, and environmental health and vitality" (Strong, 1995, p. 19; Besleme & Mullin, 1997). Similarly, the Northwest Indiana Quality of Life Council developed 75 indicators based on the concept of sustainability. The criteria that were used to select the candidate indicators and the categories into which they were organized are each associated with the concept of sustainability. For instance, every category was evaluated in terms of this guiding concept. Further, the project team selected several indicators that speak directly to the question of **carrying capacity** (i.e., the rate of use at which resources can be renewed or restored). Finally, preference was given to indicators that reflect a long-term rather than a short-term perspective.

Other initiatives have been developed on less structured bases. They are sometimes grouped under the **quality of life** heading. The federal government defines quality of life as "a general sense of happiness and satisfaction with our lives and environment. General 'quality of life' encompasses all aspects of life, including health, recreation, culture, rights, values, beliefs, aspirations, and the conditions that support a life containing these elements" (U.S. Department of Health and Human Services, 2000, p. 10). Besleme and Mullin note that quality of life indicators tend to be more focused on the short term than their counterparts, which are grounded on the *Healthy People* concept or the principle of sustainability. Many are also less concerned with the links that exist between and among indicator categories. As a result, these initiatives tend to compartmentalize indicators that pertain to economic development, health, and the environment (1997).

In a general way, the principle of sustainability can be differentiated from *Healthy People* and quality of life initiatives by its focus on the balance that exists between economic development and environmental health. This is not to say that *Healthy People* initiatives or indicators projects that are guided by the quality of life concept are antithetical to this balance. As noted above, indicators projects that are based on all three theories share much in common. In fact, their differences can be viewed primarily as a matter of foregrounding, in spite of the claims of some purists. In the case of *Healthy People* initiatives, wellness is emphasized. In the case of sustainability initiatives, the balance between economic development and environmental health is foregrounded.

In fact, the individual and collective action that follows from the development and publication of community-based indicators reports is more valuable than the indicators themselves or their guiding principles. Moreover, there is considerable evidence that indicators based on the *Healthy People* model, the principle of sustainability, and the more generic quality of life concept can each lead to positive interventions. Finally, fine distinctions among the three theories or principles cannot be drawn in a hard and fast way. Some indicators reports that include the term "quality of life" in their titles are oriented to the *Healthy People* movement; others are grounded on the concept of sustainability. Still others are based on entirely different theories, which are, nonetheless, coherent and compelling. This is certainly true with respect to the State of Vermont's indicators, which reflect a preeminent concern for the welfare of children and families.

How Will "Community" Be Defined?

Community is an imprecise term. It can refer to groupings of individuals with like interests or to geographical units. Various definitions have been used in the development of community-based indicators. The Calvert-Henderson quality of life indicators are organized at the national level (2000). The indicators developed by Northwest Environment Watch pertain to a 650,000-square-mile "super-region" that extends over the border of the United States into Canada (Strong, 1995, p. 19). The Oregon Benchmarks and Minnesota Milestones initiatives are organized at the state level (McKiernan & Plantz, 1999, p. 6). United Way of America's State of Caring Index is also organized around state-level data (2000).

Vermont elected to develop indicators at the sub-state level, but faced a challenge in doing so. Local governments in Vermont provide many of the services that are performed at the county level in other states; its 14 countries are thus relatively weak. At the same time, Vermont has no large and few medium-sized cities. As a result, the sponsors of the state's quality of life initiative decided to gather data at the school district level; Vermont has 60 school districts around which various communities of interests and identity have coalesced over time (Murphey, 1999, p. 77).

Other projects, including the Northwest Indiana initiative, have adopted the geographic foci of their metropolitan planning organizations. The Council's indicators thus pertain to Lake, Porter, and LaPorte counties, which together ring Lake Michigan's southern shore. This makes sense in Northwest Indiana because its urban core is divided among three cities. Power is diffuse in the region and strong integrating institutions are lacking. In fact, the Quality of Life Council's indicators, together with its other activities, are intended to serve this integrating function. A similar approach was adopted by the Pioneer Valley, a sub-state region that encompasses 43 cities and towns in the Connecticut River Valley in Western Massachusetts (Pioneer Valley Planning Commission, 2001). Other sets of community-based indicators, including the King County Benchmarks initiative, have been developed at the county level (Besleme & Mullin, 1997).

Community can be defined in a number of different ways. This is not to say that the definition of community that is chosen is unimportant, however. Clearly, it is. Nevertheless, no one definition of community will fit every indicators project. As is noted by Murphey: "Definitions of community should be grounded in locally-meaningful realities" (1999, p. 76).

What Categories of Measurement Will Be Adopted?

The specific categories selected will follow from the overarching theory that is chosen by the steering committee. The *Healthy People* initiative includes 28 distinct focus areas: access to quality health care; arthritis, osteoporosis, and chronic back conditions; cancer; chronic kidney disease; diabetes; disability and secondary conditions; educational and community-based programs; environmental health; family planning; food safety; health communication; heart disease and stroke; HIV; immunization and infectious diseases; injury and violence prevention; maternal, infant, and child health; medical product safety; mental health and mental disorders; nutrition and weight; occupational safety and health; oral health; physical activity and fitness; public health infrastructure; respiratory diseases; sexually transmitted diseases; substance abuse; tobacco use; and vision and hearing (Office of Disease Prevention and Health Promotion, 2000). The federal government does not recommend that a community adopt all 28 focus areas. Doing so would tax community resources and attention. A smaller set based on local needs and capacity is recommended instead. The Office of Health Prevention and Health Promotion does, however, call attention to 10 national priorities that are likely to be of concern in many communities. They pertain to the promotion of regular physical activity, healthier weight and good nutrition, the prevention and reduction of tobacco use, the prevention and reduction of substance abuse, responsible sexual behavior, mental health and well-being, safety and a reduction in violence, healthy environments, the prevention of infectious disease through immunization, and access to healthcare (2000).

Some combination of the 12 categories which are included in the Calvert-Henderson quality of life report, minus its national security indicator, are commonly adopted in the case of sustainability-based initiatives. They include education, employment, energy, the environment, health, human rights, income, infrastructure, public safety, recreation, and shelter (2000). The juxtaposition of employment and income indicators, on the one hand, and energy and environmental indicators, on the other, reflect a sustainability-based organizing principle. The indicator categories included in the Minnesota Milestones report point to the same conceptual ground (1998), as shown in Figure 6-2.

Figure 6-2 ■ Minnesota Milestone (Minnesota Milestones 1998. *Public Review Draft*)

Minnesota Milestone

Children, Families, and Learning

A. Our children will not live in poverty
B. Families will provide a stable, supportive environment for their children.
C. All children will be healthy and start school ready to learn.
D. Minnesotans will excel in basic and challenging academic skills and knowledge.

Health

E. Minnesotans will be healthy.

Community

F. Our communities will be safe, friendly, and caring.
G. People who need help providing for themselves will receive the help they need.
H. People with disabilities will participate in society.
I. People of all races, cultures, and ethnicities will be respected and participate fully in Minnesota's communities and economy.

Economic Prosperity

J. Minnesota will have sustainable, strong economic growth.
K. Minnesota's workforce will have the education and training to make the state a leader in the global economy.
L. All Minnesotans will have the economic means to maintain a reasonable standard of living.
M. All Minnesotans will have decent, safe, and affordable housing.
N. Rural areas, small cities, and urban neighborhoods throughout the state will be economically viable places for people to live and work.

Environment

O. Minnesotans will conserve natural resources to give future generations a healthy environment and a strong economy.
P. Minnesotans will improve the quality of the air, water, and earth.
Q. Minnesotans will restore and maintain healthy ecosystems that support diverse plants and wildlife.
R. Minnesotans will have opportunities to enjoy the state's natural resources.

Democracy

S. People will participate in government and politics.
T. Government in Minnesota will be cost-effective and services will be designated to meet the needs of the people who use them.

Although indicators pertaining to children and families, health, community, and democracy are included in the mix, the balance struck between five sets of indicators that pertain to economic prosperity and four sets of environmental indicators clearly serve a foundational purpose. Again, this is the hallmark of a community-based indicators report that is based on the concept of sustainability.

As is noted above, the theoretical bases of quality of life indicators are more varied than indicators that follow from either the *Healthy People* movement or the concept of sustainability. For this reason, the specific quality of life indicators that are included in a report and the manner in which they are chosen tend to be more varied in nature. Although Vermont's indicators are sometimes associated with the *Healthy Vermonter 2000* initiative, which is, in turn, associated with the federal government's *Healthy People* initiative, a concern for children and families, rather than health or sustainability, serves as its organizing principle. In this sense, it is more reflective of a quality of life approach than it is of a *Healthy People* or sustainability initiative. Nevertheless, health indicators are distributed among its 10 stated objectives; few economic or environmental indicators are employed, however (Hogan, 1999), as illustrated in Figure 6-3.

United Way of America adopted six categories that reflect a broader-based focus. Health indicators are distributed among these several categories as well, however (2000), as demonstrated in Figure 6-4.

A unique process was employed in the Hawaiian Ke Ala Hoku project to select indicator categories. Eschewing any single organizing principle,

Figure 6-3 ▪ Vermont Community Profiles (Hogan, 1999. *Vermont Communities County*)

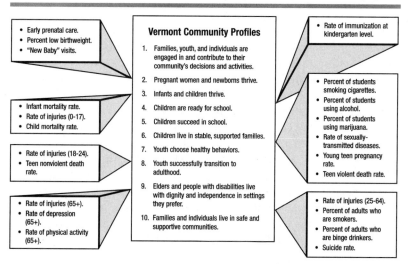

Figure 6-4 ▪ United Way State of Caring Index (United Way of America, 2000)

United Way State of Caring Index

1. Economic and financial well-being.
2. Education.
3. Health
4. Voluntarism/charity/civic engagement.
5. Safety.
6. Natural environment and other factors.

Health Indicators

- Cigarette use among 12th graders.
- Drug use among 12th graders.
- Percent low birthweight births.
- Infant mortality.
- Teen births.
- Number medically uninsured.
- Deaths per injury.

the initiative's sponsors invited 6,000 children to write about the futures that they envisioned for Hawaii. Their contributions were then distilled into a discrete set of 13 indicators (Strong, 1997, p. 19). In Marathon County, Wisconsin, focus groups were used to accomplish this same task. A total of 143 citizens participated in 10 facilitated discussions; and these same individuals were later asked to comment on the draft report that was developed (Community Planning Council of Marathon County, 1999, pp. 1–3). A list of their remarks are summarized in Box 6-1.

Although the indicator categories selected will generally follow from the underlying theory that is adopted by the steering committee (e.g., *Healthy People*, sustainability, quality of life, etc.), this discussion points to the potential value of a two- or three-theory approach. Each of the approaches described above reflects a systems perspective. Indeed, it is increasingly difficult to parse health issues from concerns pertaining to the environment and social equity issues. It is unlikely, in fact, that interventions pertaining to health, the environment, and social justice can succeed in isolation from one another, if, for no other reason, broad-based coalitions are needed to marshal public attention and resources. This suggests that a community would do well to draw on the benefits that follow from various approaches in developing their indicator categories.

Box 6-1 ■ LIFE in Marathon County, Wisconsin

1. Living a healthy life.

◆ *Percent of children up-to-date on immunizations.*

◆ *Percent of residents who use tobacco.*

◆ *Percent of residents who do not have health insurance.*

◆ *Number of individuals served through Salvation Army's noon lunch program.*

◆ *Average daily participation in National School Lunch program.*

◆ *Percent of low birthweight births.*

◆ *Percent of pregnant women receiving first trimester prenatal care.*

◆ *Number of communicable diseases reported.*

◆ *Number of preventable hospitalizations involving infants and children.*

◆ *Suicide rate.*

2. Life at school.

3. Life at work.

4. Life at leisure (the arts and recreation).

5. Life in our natural environment.

6. Living together (civics).

7. Life at home (children and families).

8. Life at home (housing).

9. Living together (public safety).

10. Living together (diversity).

What Kinds of Indicators Will Be Selected?

Three concerns pertain to this step in the development of community-based indicators. How many indicators will be developed? What specific of indicators will be chosen? How will data be gathered? Each of these questions will be addressed in turn.

Most community-based indicators reports include relatively few measures of performance in each of their several categories. This is not just due to cost; the need to focus attention is also a factor. The Pioneer Valley report thus notes: "We restricted the number of indictors we chose to track to make the report (more) easily accessible to a public that is already overloaded with information choices" (Pioneer Valley Planning Commission, 2001, p. ii). See Figure 6-5 for illustration of this process.

Select sets of measures of this kind have been called **dashboard indicators.** If every bit of information that could be provided by the computerized systems that are now integrated into our cars' various systems were, in fact, displayed on a real-time basis, we would be overwhelmed. Important information would be lost, and we would be distracted from the task at hand, that is, maneuvering our vehicle from point A to point B. Instead, we rely on a small number of indicators (i.e., speed, temperature, battery charge, etc.) that are displayed prominently on our dashboards. In the same way, a small number of community-based indicators point to the overall health of the community. They don't tell us everything we need to know. They do, however, suggest topics on which more detailed information may be required. They also enable decision makers to set priorities.

Although some indicators are common to many indicators reports, a great deal of variety is reflected in the choices that individual communities make. For instance, the Calvert-Henderson quality of life indicators address only two health concerns: infant mortality and life expectancy (2000). In contrast, United Way's State of Caring Index includes seven health-related indicators: cigarette use among 12th graders; drug use among 12th graders; percent of low birthweight births; infant mortality; teen births per 1,000 females ages 15 to 17; number of medically uninsured; and deaths per injury (2000). The Northwest Indiana Quality of Life Council's indicators report features 13 health-related measures. These

Figure 6-5 State of the Pioneer Valley Report
(Pioneer Valley Planning Commission, 2001, p. ii)

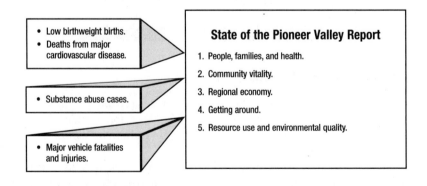

- Low birthweight births.
- Deaths from major cardiovascular disease.

- Substance abuse cases.

- Major vehicle fatalities and injuries.

State of the Pioneer Valley Report

1. People, families, and health.
2. Community vitality.
3. Regional economy.
4. Getting around.
5. Resource use and environmental quality.

several indicators are organized under two headings: "human services" and "health" (2000), as shown in Figure 6-6.

The 23 health-related indicators that are included in Vermont's community profiles pertain to early prenatal care; low birth weight births; "new baby" visits; infant mortality; rate of childhood injuries; child mortality rate; rate of full immunization; cigarette use; alcohol use; marijuana use; sexually transmitted disease; teen pregnancy; injuries among youth that result in hospitalization; violent death rate; rate of injuries resulting in hospitalization; teen death rate; injuries among elders that result in hospitalization; incidence of depression among the elderly; participation in physical activity among the elderly; adults who smoke; incidence of binge drinking; and suicide rate (Hogan, 1999). Other sets of community-based indicators include many of these same measures of community well-being and others as well. Various kinds of health-related measures are thus available to communities.

Figure 6-6 ■ Northwest Quality of Life Council Indicators Report. (Reprint with permission of Northwest Indiana Quality of Life Council, Inc.)

Northwest Indiana Quality of Life Council Indicators Report

1. Economic prosperity.
2. Environmental quality.
3. Transportation.
4. Educational excellence.
5. Human services.
6. Public safety.
7. Health.
8. Housing.
9. Recreation and tourism.
10. The arts.
11. Governance.

- Number of low birthweight births.
- Infant mortality.
- Adult and youth substance abuse rate.
- Ratio of citizens aged 80 or more to the population aged 65 or more.
- Disabled clients served as a percentage of the eligible population
- Mental health patients served as a percentage of the eligible population.

- Emergency room use for non-emergency purposes.
- Population without health insurance.
- Deaths per 100,000 due to stroke, cancer, heart disease.
- Deaths per 100,000 due to tobacco, alcohol, and other drugs.
- Total deaths per 100,000.
- AIDS cases per 100,000.
- Median cost of healthcare as a percent of median income.

One final caution must be noted with respect to the selection of indicators. Historically, chambers of commerce and other business and civic organizations have gathered and publicized positive data about their communities. They seek new residents, businesses, and the jobs and investment dollars that they bring. In contrast, the focus of the contemporary community-based indicators movement is problem-solving. This means that unflattering data must be gathered and shared as well. As a result, "disparities at sub-levels" may come to light, much to the consternation of some business and political leaders (Murphey, 1999, p. 77).

To a certain extent, these kinds of concerns can be alleviated by involving business and political leaders in the planning process. Additionally, the use of explanatory notes can relieve fears that data will be misused (Murphey, 1999, p. 77). Finally, engaging community leaders in problem-solving activities can help to overcome objections. In this way, business and political leaders can be afforded the opportunity to draw attention to the contributions that they are making to an improved quality of life rather than to blame for past performance.

Once a select set of indicators is chosen, appropriate data can be gathered. As is noted above, a great deal of information is available from extant sources. Using these sources reduces costs. It also provides benchmarks against which comparisons can be made. Census data is featured prominently in almost all community-based indicators reports. Many other federal agencies gather and maintain data for more specialized purposes. For instance, the *Healthy People* initiative relies on data derived from the National Center for Health Statistics' National Health and Nutrition Survey, National Health Interview Survey, and National Survey of Family Growth. It also uses data obtained from the Substance Abuse and Mental Health Services Administration's National Household Survey on Drug Abuse and other federal sources (U.S. Department of Health and Human Services, 2000). The Pioneer Valley indicators report cites the Bureau of Economic Analysis' Regional Economic Information System and the Department of Agriculture's Agricultural Census (Pioneer Valley Planning Commission, 2001). United Way of America's State of Caring Index makes use of data secured from the Justice Department's Bureau of Justice Statistics and the Federal Election Commission (United Way of America, 2000). In fact, the federal government gathers and publishes data on a broad range of demographic, economic, environmental, health, housing, public safety, and social concerns.

State and local governmental sources are also used. The Vermont initiative relies heavily on data gathered and maintained by various state agencies (Murphey, 1999, p. 77). The Marathon County report uses data secured from the Wisconsin Department of Public Instruction, the coroner's office, and the local Health Department (Community Planning

Council of Marathon County, 1999). Similarly, the Pioneer Valley initiative draws on data maintained by the Massachusetts Department of Revenue, the State Board of Education, the Massachusetts Department of Public Health, and the State Police (Pioneer Valley Planning Commission, 2001). Data pertaining to transportation is available from the metropolitan planning organizations that serve most regions in the country. Data concerning the environment and economic development is gathered and maintained by many of these same entities as well.

Private-sector sources of information, including both nonprofit organizations and research institutes, are also used. The Marathon County initiative secures data from the Salvation Army and the local United Way affiliate (Community Planning Council of Marathon County, 1999). To supplement its own data, the United Way of America initiative draws on data gathered and maintained by the Independent Sector and the National Center for Charitable Statistics (United Way of America, 2000).

Some indicators initiatives supplement these kinds of data with local surveys. Despite the cost, a survey may be appropriate when local perceptions pertaining to such issues as racial diversity, social justice, and satisfaction with public services are deemed to be of critical importance. Alternatively, focus groups can be conducted using questions derived from an analysis of readily available data. Discussion summaries or transcripts can then be analyzed, and findings can be incorporated into the narrative sections of indicators reports (Krueger, 1997).

What Kinds of Comparisons Will Be Made?

Data presented without context convey little meaning. This fact can be illustrated in the old joke about the conversation between a doctor and a client. After a thorough examination, the client says: "Tell it to me straight doc. I can take it. How long have I got?" The doctor replies: "Eight." The anxious client then asks: "What do you mean, doc? Eight years? Eight months? Eight weeks?" The doctor looks at his watch and proceeds to count down: "Seven, six, five . . ."

Context is important. In the case of community-based indicators, points of comparison are essential. Typically, one, two, or three points of comparison are made: performance can be assessed against a community's own performances in prior time periods; performances can be assessed against an established target or goal; and performance can be assessed against the performances of other communities. The relative merits of each approach will be examined in turn.

Trend data is often reported using charts and graphs. The display of raw numbers is recommended as well, however, so that a reader can conduct his or her own analysis. Three-year, five-year, and ten-year comparisons are often employed in indicators reports. The chief advantage of multiple data points, of course, is that they facilitate the identification of patterns (e.g., long-term trends, cyclical swings, and temporary aberrations).

In some cases, simple but effective techniques can be used to call attention to certain trends. The State of the Pioneer Region report includes a "thumbs up" or "thumb-down" symbol next to all five of its indicator categories as well as each of 14 indicators (2001). The symbols signify whether performances are trending up or down. United Way of America uses a similar approach in its State of Caring Index. Arrows show whether national performance has improved, declined, or remained steady or reflected mixed trends over the ten-year period ending in 1998. A total of 17 indicators reflect improving trends (i.e., median household income, population below poverty, unemployment rate, home affordability, math scores, reading scores, science scores, public school expenditures, pupil-teacher ratios, injury-related death rate, births to teen mothers, infant mortality rate, nonprofit financial ratios, percentage that volunteer, property crime, violent crime, and safe air); another 12 show declining trends (i.e., income inequality, renter affordability, writing scores, medically uninsured people, children with a single parent, low birthweight babies, hard drug use in high school, cigarette use in high school, average hours volunteered, community giving, voter turnout, and traffic delays during peak periods); and three indicators reflect steady or mixed trends (i.e., high school dropouts, teacher salaries, and safe water) (2000, p. 11).

A comparison against a target or goal can also be effective, particularly when combined with trend data. In fact, three benefits can accrue from the use of targets or goals. First, it can prompt decision makers to envision a better future. The following kinds of questions can thus be posed. What high school dropout rate is the community ready to accept? What is an acceptable immunization rate for children? Given the relationship that exists between air quality and economic activity, how much air pollution is the community willing to tolerate? And what level of voting is indicative of a vibrant civic life? Answering these kinds of questions can lead to the development of a collective vision for a community. Second, goals and targets are needed if priorities are to be established. Although community-specific data that is tracked over time can contribute to discussions of this kind, a trend line that advances forever is not necessarily "good." Conversely, a trend line that dips on occasion is not necessarily "bad." Priorities depend on such factors as an indicator's "criticality," its distance from an established goal or target, and its relationship to other indicators. This kind of information is difficult to divine from trend data. In fact, it requires an ongoing conversation among the many elements that make up a diverse community. Third, goals and targets facilitate tracking over time. Progress—or lack thereof—can be best assessed against an established benchmark (Besleme & Mullin, 1997).

The health-related targets adopted in the *Healthy People* movement illustrate each of these three benefits. Elements of a collective vision pertaining to health are embedded in the presentation of each of the initiative's 467 indicators. For instance, one indicator calls attention to the fact that 43 percent of the population now lives in federally designated ozone non-attainment areas. The target for 2010 is zero percent. Another indicator shows that 65 percent of nonsmokers are routinely exposed to environmental tobacco smoke. The goal for 2010 is 45 percent (U.S. Department of Health and Human Services, 2000, p. 40). In this way, the *Healthy People* movement reflects a larger vision for the nation. Further, the initiative's objectives were established in a collective fashion. The Healthy People Consortium is a coalition of some 350 national organizations and over 250 state and local units of government. Additionally, two requests for input generated over 11,000 comments (U.S. Department of Health and Human Services, 2000). Finally, the *Healthy People* initiative calls on local communities to develop action plans that can lead to improved performances in select sets of indicators. In each of these ways, the Healthy People initiative illustrates the value of comparisons to established goals or targets.

Comparisons over time and against goals and targets are used in most community-based indicators reports. Community-to-community performances tend to be more problematic. Some steering committees eschew the "natural human tendency (perhaps taken to new heights in our culture) to want to ask (and want to answer) the question, 'who's better, who's worse?' or even 'who's best, who's worst?'" (Murphey, 1999, p. 79). Others believe that comparisons of this kind can spur positive action. United Way of America's State of Caring Index clearly reflects this alternative view. It ranks every state in the Union in 32 indicators that are organized into six broad categories. Further, it weighs and then indexes the results on a 1,000-point scale. Indices often require the use of weights, since it is unlikely that all indicators will be perceived to be of equal importance. This can put strains on the kinds of coalitions that are sometimes involved in developing community-based indicators. For instance, it cannot be assumed that the environmental community and public health officials will agree on the appropriate weights to be assigned to indicators pertaining to water quality and immunization levels. The use of indices can thus heighten political sensibilities. Further, business and political leaders whose communities are likely to fall into the bottom quartile of an index cannot be expected to welcome the publication of this kind of data.

Respectively, the six indicators in the "economic and financial well-being" category are worth 24 percent of the index's total value; the eight indictors of the "education" category, the eight indicators of the "health" category, and the five indicators of the "volunteerism/charity/civic engagement" category are each worth 20 percent of the index's 1,000 points; the two indictors in the "safety" category account for 10 percent of the index's total value; and the three indicators in the "natural environment and other factors" category account for the remaining 6 percent of the index's 1,000 points. The index thus permits comparisons between states. Data for the year 2000 indicates that Minnesota had the best overall performance among the 50 states, achieving a score of 701. The lowest score was 298 (2000). This kind of comparison is clearly intended to spur action at both the state and local levels.

The State of Vermont has adopted a middle position between these two views. School-district level data is not published in the indicators report, but assistance is provided to communities that choose to make their own comparisons (Murphey, 1999, p. 79). This approach is recommended, together with comparisons over time and against established goals or objectives.

What Kind of Background Information Will Accompany the Data?

Most sets of indicators are compiled into reports, copies of which are made available both electronically and in a hard copy format. Typically, community-based indicators reports include background information about the theory that guided the initiative. An extensive discussion of the concept of sustainability is thus reflected in the Northwest Indiana Quality of Life Council's indicators report (2000). Other reports describe the *Healthy People* initiative.

Explanations as to why certain categories and indicators were selected are often provided as well. The LIFE in Marathon County report thus includes a paragraph under the heading "Why Are We Concerned?" for each indicator. The explanation for a performing arts attendance indicator thus reads: "Performing arts events, including music, dance, and drama, provide entertainment and a means of broadening cultural horizons. Healthy attendance at performing arts events enriches that aspect of the quality of life which focuses on the arts and entertainment" (Community Planning Council of Marathon County, 1999, p. 46). The introduction to the "economy and financial well-being" category of the United Way of America's State of Caring Index notes that "Economic resources and opportunities have a fundamental impact on peoples' lives. For this reason, economic factors have been heavily weighted in the index. Clearly, poverty greatly disadvantages a significant portion of our population and adversely affects most of the other indicators" (United Way of America, 2000, p. 4). Although brief, this commentary reminds the reader of the United Way's systematic approach and sets the stage for a description of the indicators that follow. Reflecting another strategy, an interpretive essay accompanies each of the 12 sections of the Calvert-Henderson quality of life indicators report (2000).

How Will the Indictors Be Used?

McKiernan and Plantz draw a sharp distinction between **community status reports** and **community interventions** (1999). In doing so, they recognize that it is necessary, first, to develop a set of community-based indicators reports. In and of themselves, however, community-based indicators—no matter how well-developed—cannot produce action; they can only serve as catalysts for change. Besleme and Mullin thus note that "The belief that indicators, in and of themselves, can mobilize change in our nation's communities is one that we must disavow" (1997). Whereas indicators reports provide information about community conditions, interventions "change selected conditions in the community." Further, the selection of "conditions of interest" serves as a starting point in the development of indicators reports. In contrast, **community interventions** begin with the identification of desired outcomes (McKiernan & Plantz, 1999).

McKiernan and Plantz (1999) identify four steps that are essential to community interventions: (1) a comprehensive plan for achieving specified outcomes is developed; (2) a detailed action plan is prepared; (3) specific indicators that show the extent to which outcomes and milestones are being achieved are selected; and (4) an implementation plan for measuring achievement is developed and implemented.

In Marathon County, Wisconsin, 11 priorities were established based on the 77 indicators that were included in its LIFE in Marathon County report. They pertain to child care, affordable housing, alcohol and drug use, discrimination and acceptance of diversity, family abuse, health insurance coverage, poverty and insufficient income, preventive health care, water quality, youth at risk, and public safety. Three types of information are provided with respect to each priority: (1) the indicators against which performance will be tracked; (2) specific actions that are being taken or will be taken; and (3) a narrative assessment of progress. Seven indicators are thus cited with respect to the preventive health care priority: childhood immunizations; tobacco use; low birth weight births; suicide rate; prenatal care; communicable diseases; and lead poisoning. With respect to "action," the report notes that "The Regional Early Childhood Immunization

Network is a centralized database that assists in analyzing childhood immunization rates and reminding families when their child's immunizations are due. There has been an increase in funding devoted to raising awareness (about the need) to increase the number of children screened for lead poisoning. Grants provide support and services that aim to reduce the incidence of low-birthweight (births)." With respect to "progress," the report concludes: "Indicators reveal that significant progress has been made on lead poisoning, low-birthweight (births), and childhood immunization rates in 1999. Recent preventive care measures have led to improvements (that suggest we are making) progress toward our goals" (Community Planning Council of Marathon County, 1999, p. 13). Although some readers may desire more detailed information, the structure of Marathon County's action report should be considered a model. Specific indicators are tied to specific actions, which, in turn, are assessed on an ongoing basis.

Community interventions can be organized in at least three ways. The most proactive involves the formation of a standing committee or task force to address each priority that is selected. Invitations are issued to representatives of governmental agencies, private-sector organizations, and other parties who have an interest in the subject. The committee or task force meets on a regular basis. Its work is sanctioned by the umbrella organization that developed and published the community-based indicators report. An action plan is then developed and pursued.

Less proactive interventions can also be beneficial. In Northwest Indiana, the Quality of Life Council uses its indicators report to select topics to be addressed in an ongoing series of quarterly meetings to which decision makers representing various sectors of the community are invited. An "expert" is typically asked to give a presentation on a particular topic. This is followed by an open discussion, which, in turn, leads either to the adoption of a resolution or the sanctioning of an ad hoc team to further study the issue and develop a set of recommendations to be directed to appropriate actors in the region. Besleme and Mullin testify to the potential value of this more passive use of indicators. "The influence of information is almost always indirect, and it may take a fair amount of time before the information becomes manifested in actions, initiatives, or policy agendas. In terms of inspiring debate, however, both healthy communities and community indicators have demonstrated that goals can be set in a way that leads to community change" (1997).

In the least proactive approach, existing organizations are called upon to incorporate the priorities established in the final phase of a community-based indicators initiative into their own strategic and tactical plans. A Health Department might thus be challenged to develop a plan to reduce gun violence to a level identified in an indictors report. Similarly, local units of government might be asked to develop a land use plan that has the potential of achieving a population density target established in a community status report. This approach can also be used in conjunction with the standing committee or task force model and the "resolutions" model.

A cautionary note must attend to each of these models. Indicators can be useful in identifying a community's strengths and weaknesses. They can also engender the public's attention and contribute to the development of priorities. The link between a specific indicator and a particular outcome cannot be assumed, however. This is so for at least two reasons: (1) there may be little or no correlation between a particular indicator and a desired outcome; and (2) an indicator may produce both positive and negative outcomes. An example of the first concern is illustrated in a study reported by Kanarek and his colleagues (2000). Using survey data, the researchers examined the relationship between selected health status indicators, including various demographic, health, and socioeconomic data, and reports of "ill health." Together, the indicators accounted for about 11 percent of the variability in reported unhealthy days. Socioeconomic and health-related factors accounted for virtually all of the variability, however; age, population size, and population density were not found to be related to subjective reports of health. On its face, the study's finding confounds the kind of shared thinking that can spur the development of community-based indicators. Many people undoubtedly believe that population density is positively related to ill health. After all, high population density exposes individuals to higher levels of air pollution and stress producers such as high-volume traffic and increased criminal activity. At the same time, however, the residents of large cities may enjoy access to higher quality health care and high-paying jobs that are harder to find in rural settings. The relationship between an indicator and a particular health outcome can thus be complex. For this reason, research is needed to establish the precise relationships that exist between specific indicators and any set of outcomes that are identified.

As noted above, research is also needed because particular indicators may reflect both positive and negative outcomes. This is less of a problem in the case of indicators that are based on the *Healthy People* initiative than it is in the case of some indicators that are based on the concept of sustainability. This is so because the term "sustainability" embodies a dynamic tension that exists between economic activity and environmental health. As was noted above, housing starts can be viewed both positively and negatively. In the short term, new construction can bring jobs to a community. At the same time, housing starts can reflect the kind of suburban sprawl that is antithetical to a community's vision for itself. Again, statistical analysis, benchmarking, and other forms of research that are tied to the community's vision can contribute positively to the development of indicators and their use.

This cautionary note in no way undermines the potential value of community-based indicators or the community interventions that a report can engender. Complex economic, environmental, and social concerns are addressed in initiatives of this kind. Multifaceted relationships are arrayed across several very different domains. Further, an effective intervention requires the engagement of many actors, some of whom may harbor very different perceptions of a particular priority and how it should be approached. In this sense, a community-based indicators report should be viewed as a starting point; it cannot serve as the culmination of an initiative. At best, it can provide a foundation on which a research agenda can be constructed and action plans can be developed.

How Will the Indicators Be Maintained?

Data changes over time. So, too, do community priorities. For these reasons, community-based indicators need to be updated on a regular basis. This includes the theory that served as a foundation for the original report, the indicator categories that were employed, the kinds of data that were gathered with respect to each indicator, and the data sources that were used. A review of this kind should also be accompanied by formal evaluations of any interventions that were undertaken following the publication of the most recent indicators report. Most important, a review of certain indicators can facilitate a reassessment of community priorities. It can also provide another opportunity to mobilize public attention.

Both the Northwest Indiana Quality of Life Council and the Planning Council of Marathon County update their indicators on a biannual basis (Community Planning Council of Marathon County, 1999, p. 11). This time frame is recommended. Trends can become evident over the course of two years. The progress of a community intervention—or lack thereof—can also become apparent within this time frame.

In this way, community-based indicators and the interventions that they engender can echo the four societal trends that were noted in the first section of this chapter. They can come to reflect a sophisticated understanding of human flourishing. Further, they can serve to reveal the complex relationships that exist among the many factors that contribute to a high quality of life. Community-based indicators can also contribute to the development of what Benjamin Barber refers to as strong democracy. Finally, they can reflect a community's commitment to continuous improvement, that is, the iterative use of data to improve work processes. For each of these reasons, it is important that a community-based indicators initiative not be viewed as a one-time effort. It is part and parcel of what it means for a community to flourish over time in all of its many dimensions.

 KEY POINTS

- The development of community-based indicators and community interventions is linked to four larger societal trends: (1) the on-going development of our understanding of the concept of human flourishing; (2) a new appreciation for the systematic nature of the many factors that contribute to a high quality of life; (3) an increasing reorientation to the concerns of local community; and (4) a growing recognition of the community's need to commit to continuous improvement.

- Need for adequate funding and several different funding alternatives should be examined when planning indicator initiatives.

- Three theories or sets of principles together, undergird most community-based indicators initiatives (i.e., the *Healthy People* movement, the principle of sustainability, and the quality of life concept).

- Several different conceptions of the term "community" should be considered; no one definition is appropriate for every indicators initiative.

- Different sets of indicator categories should be compared and contrasted.

- There are a number of concerns pertaining to the selection and development of individual indicators, including the number to be selected and the kinds of data sources that can be employed.

- There are advantages and disadvantages of the three kinds of comparisons (i.e., against a community's own performance over time, against a target or goal, and against the performances of other communities). The first two are recommended; the third is not.

- There are specific kinds of kinds of narrative data that typically accompany indicator categories and individual measures in indicator reports.

- There are three ways in which indicators can be employed in community interventions; they range from the very proactive to the much less proactive.

- Indicators need to be updated on a regular basis.

REFERENCES

Barber, B. R. (1984). *Strong democracy: Participatory politics for a new age.* Los Angeles: University of California Press.

Besleme, K., & Mullin, M. (1997). Community indicators and healthy communities. *National Civic Review, 86,* 43–52.

Block, P. (1987). *The empowered manager: Positive political skills at work.* San Francisco: Jossey-Bass Publishers.

Community Planning Council. (1999). *LIFE in Marathon County.*

Covey, S. R. (1989). *The seven habits of highly effective people.* New York: Simon and Schuster.

Deming, W. E. (1986). *Out of the crisis.* Cambridge, MA: Massachusetts Institute of Technology.

Handy, C. (1998). *The hungry spirit: Beyond capitalism, a quest for purpose in the modern world.* New York: Broadway Books.

Held, D. (1995). *Democracy and the global order.* Stanford, CA: Stanford University Press.

Henderson, H., Lickerman, J., & Flynn, P. (Eds.). (2000). *Calvert-Henderson quality of life indicators.* Bethesda, MD: Calvert Group, Ltd.

Hogan, C. D. (1999). *Vermont Communities County.*

International Council for Local Environmental Initiatives. (1996). *The Local Agenda 21 Planning Guide.*

Juran, J. M. (Ed.). (1974). *Juran's quality control handbook.* New York: McGraw-Hill.

Kanarek, N. (2000). Community indicators of health-related quality of life—United States, 1993–1997. *Journal of the American Medical Association, 283,* 2097–2099.

Kast, F., & Rosenzweig, J. A. (1972). General systems theory: Applications for organization and management. *Academy of Management Journal,* 447–465.

Katz, D., & Kahn, R. L. (1966). *The social psychology of organizations.* New York: John Wiley and Sons.

Krueger, R. A. (1997). *Analyzing and reporting focus group results.* Thousands Oaks, CA: Sage.

Lowery, D. (2001). Implementing quality programs in the not-for-profit sector: The role of intermediaries. *Quality Progress, 34,* 75–80.

McKiernan, L. C., & Plantz, M. C. (1999). Community report cards and targeted community interventions. *Community 2,* 6–12.

Minnesota Milestones. (1998). *Public Review Draft.*

Moore, T. (1992). *Care of the soul.* New York: Harper-Collins.

Murphey, D. A. (1999). Presenting community-level data in an 'outcomes and indicators' framework: Lessons from Vermont's experience. *Public Administration Review, 59,* 76–82.

Northwest Indiana Quality of Life Council. (2000). *Northwest Indiana Quality of Life Indicators.*

Office of Disease Prevention and Health Promotion. (2001). *Healthy people in healthy communities: A community planning guide using Healthy People 2010.* Washington, DC: U.S. Government Printing Office.

Oregon Progress Board. (1999). *Redefining progress.*

Payne, D. (2000). *Evaluating service-learning activities and programs.* Lanham, MD: Scarecrow.

Pioneer Valley Planning Commission. (2001). *State of the pioneer valley.*

President's Council on Sustainable Development. (1996). *Sustainable America: A new consensus for prosperity, opportunity, and a healthy environment for the future.* Washington, DC: U.S. Government Printing Office.

Strong, S. (1995). Link block grants to quality-of-life measures. *Christian Science Monitor, 87,* 19.

Strong, S. (1997). The link between quality of data and quality of life. *Christian Science Monitor, 89,* 19.

United Way of America. (1996). *Measuring program outcomes: A practical approach.*

United Way of America. (2000). *State of Caring Index.*

U.S. Department of Health and Human Services. (2000). *Healthy People 2010: Understanding and improving health.* Washington, DC: U.S. Government Printing Office.

Chapter

7

ANALYZING INDICATORS
AND USING THE ANALYSIS
C. David Strupeck

 LEARNING OBJECTIVES

At the conclusion of the chapter, the reader will be able to:

- ◆ Conduct the final step in the Ontario Needs Impact Based Model, analysis of the information.
- ◆ Describe the steps in the scientific method of research.
- ◆ Describe a variety of research methods, tools, and techniques.
- ◆ Identify the steps in a grant proposal.
- ◆ Write an action plan that includes a request for proposal and a proposal review process.

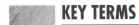 **KEY TERMS**

Action plan	Request for proposal (RFP)
Action steps	Scientific method
Analysis	Statistical Package for
Delphi method	the Social Sciences (SPSS)
QSR NVivo	Survey

T his chapter delves into the myriad tasks necessary to accomplish the overall objective of increasing the quality of life in our communities. The tasks discussed here are included in step four of the Ontario Needs Impact Based Model, the processing and analysis of the information gathered during the first three steps. The tasks are many and, at times, may seem unrelated. All work will eventually lead to a plan of action to achieve improvement in the health of the community. Along the way, we will briefly visit a variety of topics, including research methodology and methods, tools and techniques, and proposals. Additionally, examples of previous community assessment research will be presented as part of the action plan.

Analysis of the data gathered during the needs assessment process depends in large part on the nature of the information gathered. For example, we have previously discussed the use of focus groups. The information gathered from these groups is analyzed much differently from that garnered by using a survey with Likert scales. The uses of the findings also depend on the information gathered and the analysis of the data. If we find that a particular community has, for example, experienced 20 stroke deaths per 100,000 population and *Healthy People 2010* has a goal of 48 stroke deaths per 100,000, this then allows us to focus on other community needs since the current rate is lower than the target rate.

Ultimately, the analysis should help us determine which community needs require the most attention. The group sponsoring the needs assessment will need to prioritize the findings and begin the process of how the needs should be addressed. The process of prioritizing can be difficult, as we cannot be all things to all people and solve all problems within the context of one targeted solution.

ANALYSIS OF THE INFORMATION

Analysis is the study and examination of data. The fourth step in the Ontario Needs Impact Based Model requires analysis of the data gathered during the first three steps of the model. Analysis is necessary to determine comparative needs of the community relative to *Healthy People 2010*. The analysis may reveal patterns and or trends in the well-being of the community.

The steps in the analysis process include categorization, summarization, comparison, and inference. Box 7-1 illustrates one way by which a community needs assessment may present an analysis.

Box 7-1 ■ Northwest Indiana Community Health Needs Assessment

---

Category: Healthy People 2010 (Goal 9): Improve pregnancy planning and spacing and prevent unintended pregnancy.

Objective: Reduce pregnancies among adolescent females to 46 pregnancies per 1000.

Data: Gary, Indiana has one of the highest adolescent pregnancy rates in the United States (Ishmael, 1999). 1 out of 25 adolescents 15-17 years old in Lake County will become pregnant. If they drop out of school, and 80 percent do, 1 out of 4 will be pregnant again within a year (Indiana State Department of Health, Epidemiological Resource Center, 1996).

Summary: Current rate in Lake County is 40 per 1000 plus 25 percent of the 32 that drop out of school results in a rate of 48 per 1000.

Comparison: Lake County rate is 48 versus Healthy People 2010 target rate of 46.

Inference: Lake County needs some improvement; find rate for Gary, Indiana. If rate in Gary is inordinately high, decreasing the pregnancy rate in Gary would decrease the rate in Lake County to the Healthy People 2010 target.

A BRIEF OVERVIEW OF THE SCIENTIFIC METHOD

Research is basically a systematic search for truth. The operative term here is systematic, that is, following a step-by-step process that is valid, reliable, and able to be replicated. The steps in the **scientific method** are:

1. Clearly identify and state the problem
2. State the research hypothesis (es)
3. Determine information needs and gather data
4. Process data and test the hypothesis (es)
5. State the findings

Along the way, documentation is necessary. The documentation needs to be written in a clear, grammatically correct, unambiguous fashion. The statement, "Too many adults with high blood pressure," is not as clear as the statement, "The incidence of adults with high blood pressure in *our community* is 29.8 percent while the HP 2010 objective is 16 percent." If we observe the systematic steps in the scientific method, our needs assessment has a greater chance of accomplishing the end objective of healthier communities.

RESEARCH METHODS

There are innumerable ways by which we can gather and analyze data. The following tools, techniques, and methods will be explained and discussed:

1. The Survey method
2. The Delphi method
3. SPSS
4. QSR NVivo
5. Descriptive statistics

The Survey Method

One way that we can collect information about the world or a community is through use of a **survey.** This method is appropriate if we are able to ask people questions in a standardized format, cannot contact the total population, and yet wish to generalize findings to that population and other methods, such as case studies, are not feasible. The survey instrument must be well written, containing well-thought-out questions, and must be administered in a standardized fashion that results in valid and reliable data, permitting analysis and generalization to the population.

Once the survey instrument has been designed and tested, the survey sample must be selected. Questions regarding size of the sample, randomness, and expected response rate must be answered. Returned instruments must be coded and the data entered into a computer program, such as SPSS (more later).

The Delphi Method

The Rand Corporation devised the **Delphi method** in the 1950s (Dalkey & Hemer, 1963) as a means to handle opinions rather than objective facts. We must first identify a group of experts who agree to participate in a series of ranking-type surveys. Through an iterative process, the experts are asked to provide their opinions on a gradually shrinking set of concepts in an effort to reach a consensus within the group. There are two very important issues that need to be resolved when using the Delphi approach (Schmidt, 1997). First, when do we stop polling the experts? Too soon risks less meaning for the rankings, while too many risks wasting the time of the experts, resulting in some dropouts. Second, how many items should be carried forward from each round? Too many items can cause confusion and delay consensus, while too few may prematurely eliminate important items.

This method appears to be especially appropriate to the health care profession and is used frequently. The National Institute for Occupational Safety and Health (NIOSH) used a consensus building process in 1998 to set priorities during the next decade for occupational and health research (Rosenstock, Olenec & Wagner, 1998). Abbott Laboratories (as reported by Blair et al., 1996) sponsored the Facing the Uncertain Future project, which is managed and administered by the Medical Group Management Association (MGMA) and the American College of Medical Practice Executives (ACPME). In addition, research findings suggest that Delphi groups outperform statistical groups and standard interacting groups (Rowe & Wright, 1999).

Statistical Package for the Social Sciences (SPSS)

There are many methods by which we are able to analyze data. One is through the use of statistical computerized software packages. The **statistical package for the social sciences (SPSS)** is one such package. Data entered via the data editor in SPSS provides a convenient way in which we can create data files and subsequently analyze the data. The data editor makes it easy to label variables, define missing values, and modify display formats. This software is readily available at a variety of prices, depending on the size of the sample. Many university bookstores sell a student version (small sample sizes) while a comprehensive license for the software is available from SPSS Inc. (Chicago, IL). Ideally, the community team should include a university professor with SPSS expertise on the coalition team. That individual should be able to obtain and apply the software for the community needs assessment and analysis.

QSR NVivo

QSR NVivo is a software program for qualitative analysis. It provides ways of managing data and developing and exploring ideas that would not be possible if we were using paper and index cards. Qualitative analysis usually requires that we explore and interpret messy data, such as interviews (focus groups), documents, and field notes. These methods are designed to capture life as participants live it or see it, rather than fit responses into categories designed by a researcher. Fox and Roberts (1999) studied written comments from a group of MDs using list serve technology. Doctors could send messages to the list, which were automatically sent via email to the other doctors, whose replies would also be circulated to the list. Roberts actually became an active member of the group and posed questions to the MDs as he and Fox tried to develop explanations for what they observed in this virtual community. The data analyzed was all text—no counts, no frequencies, no or other quantities.

These types of research methods are most often used when the investigator is looking for explanations, descriptions, or evaluations of life or some microcosm of society. The analysis of this type of data can be painstakingly slow. NVivo is designed to allow researchers to enter their notes into a program, even coding the text during entry. This allows researchers to manipulate and find specific text without having to sort through page after page of notes or index cards. NVivo is an entirely new program, very different from its predecessors NUD*IST4 and N5. It is designed for researchers using rich text data requiring fine-detailed methods of analysis (Richards, 1999).

Descriptive Statistics

Many researchers today are enamored of inferential statistics, which are used to estimate how likely it is that a statistical result based on data from a random sample is representative of the population from which the sample is assumed to have been selected. Generalizations from sample research require the use of such tools. However, we should not overlook a rather simple, yet revealing, tool such as **descriptive statistics.** For example, one research study tested data for statistically significant differences between return on investment (ROI) using foreign accounting practices versus ROI for the same firms' annual reports using U.S. accounting practices (Rueschhoff & Strupeck, 1998). No statistical significance was found, yet the authors discovered an overall difference in ROI of 3.4 percent between foreign and U.S. accounting practices, which most investors would consider important. Would you rather invest your money in a fund that returned ten percent or a fund that returned 13.4 percent? In business, we call this a no brainer, yet the inferential statistical tools used (which were appropriate given the data) in the above study did not allow the authors to state that there was a difference between the accounting practices.

Community assessment projects can be well served with descriptive statistics. Measures of central tendency, such as means, medians, and modes, may be very telling when considering the overall health of a community. The mean represents the average of a data distribution, the median is the point that divides the distribution in half, and the mode is the most frequent value(s) in the distribution. Consider the data range shown in Table 7-1. The mean is $68,533, the median (#17) is $68,125, and the mode is $65,000.

Simple frequency tables, available through SPSS or Microsoft Excel, may reveal important differences between *Healthy People 2010* objectives and community data. Figure 7-1 shows a frequency distribution from a descriptive Internet study conducted by the National Geographic Society. The statements that correspond to the chart are as follows:

Complex: The world is too complex for me.

Belong: I don't feel I belong to anything I'd call a community.

Favor: People who do a favor expect nothing in return.

Valuable: I have something valuable to give to the world.

Better World: The world is becoming a better place for everyone.

As the bar chart indicates, the statement receiving the most positive response during the survey was the one addressing personal self-worth (87.4 percent agreed with the statement). Given the phrasing of the other statements, all received more positive than negative responses but not as overwhelmingly as the "valuable" statement. For example, 65.3 percent disagreed with the negatively phrased statement, "I don't feel I belong to anything I'd call a community," thereby indicating that more of the respondents believed they did belong than those who felt that they did not belong to a community.

TABLE 7-1 Income Distribution

ID	EDUCATION	SALARY
1	15	$80,000
2	17	$78,500
3	18	$78,250
4	19	$78,125
5	19	$75,000
6	19	$75,000
7	18	$73,750
8	19	$73,500
9	19	$72,500
10	19	$70,875
11	19	$70,000
12	16	$70,000
13	20	$69,250
14	19	$68,750
15	17	$68,750
16	18	$68,125
17	19	$68,125
18	17	$67,500
19	18	$66,875
20	19	$66,875
21	16	$66,750
22	19	$66,250
23	16	$66,000
24	21	$65,000
25	17	$65,000
26	19	$65,000
27	18	$62,500
28	19	$61,875
29	19	$61,875
30	19	$61,250
31	16	$60,625
32	19	$60,375
33	16	$60,000
Total		$2,262,250

Figure 7-1 ■ Frequency of Agreement/Disagreement of Respondents' Views on the World, Its Inhabitants, and Its Future
(Source: http://survey2000.nationalgeographic.com/community.html)

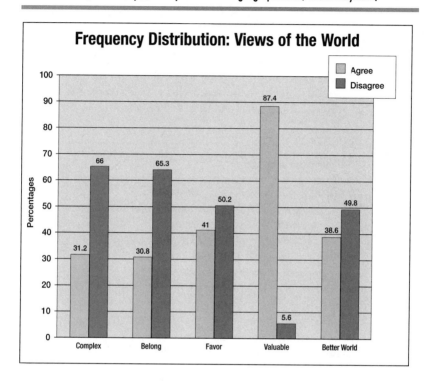

Using simple percentages may also reveal some interesting information. The goals of *Healthy People 2010* are stated as percentages of the population. For example, Goal 1: "Improve access to comprehensive, high-quality health care services," has as one objective "increasing the proportion of persons with health insurance from a baseline of 86% covered by health insurance in 1997 to 100% coverage." Data collected by the community needs assessment team in Northwest Indiana revealed that "28% of adults making less than $15,000 per year, 29% of adults making between $15,000 and $18,000, and 22% making between $20,000 and $24,000 do not have health insurance coverage." We can readily observe that, in Indiana, in these income brackets, these members of the community represent a greater percentage than the 14 percent of U.S. citizens who did not have health insurance in 1997.

GRANT PROPOSALS

Eventually, the community needs assessment process will lead to prioritized needs, necessitating funding to address research and projects specifically regarding these needs. There are innumerable funding sources for community health projects. All require completion of a grant proposal, given the **request for proposal (RFP)**.

A sample outline for proposals is presented in Box 7-2 (Tornquist, 1986). Obviously, a great deal of work is required to prepare such a document. This outline enables the researchers to tell potential funding sources why, how, and to what end they will do a study.

Box 7-2 ■ Grant Proposal Outline

I. *Introduction and review of the literature*
  A. *The problem needing a solution, the question to be answered, or the theory to be tested*
  B. *The work already done or prior tests of the theory*
  C. *Gaps or shortcomings in the work done to date*
  D. *The purpose of the present study*
II. *Methods*
  A. *The design of the study*
  B. *Setting and sample*
  C. *Intervention, if applicable*
  D. *Variables and their measurement*
  E. *Research procedures*
III. *Plans for analysis and use*
  A. *The data expected*
  B. *Types of analyses planned*
  C. *Uses of the outcomes*
  D. *Limitations of the study*

If the action plan includes RFPs that address the comparative needs identified by the coalition team, a procedure for disseminating, receiving, and ranking submitted RFPs must be designed. Establishing and adhering to time frames is important. The ranking guidelines should be part of the RFP so interested parties address the team's priorities and focus for the proposals. The proposal review process should adhere to the guidelines and the time frame established before the RFP is distributed to the community.

The key elements for the review process are:

1. Identification of the priority of the comparative needs
2. Specific areas of action/research to be conducted by the grantees
3. A time frame for submission of the proposals to the coalition team
4. A time frame for review of the submitted proposals
5. A system of quantifying the submitted proposals, for example, ranking by importance, focus on comparative needs, breadth of impact, and so on
6. A time frame for announcing acceptable RFPs

Figure 7-2 is a sample RFP checklist and rating form (Nardi et al., 2000), which could be used in step 5 above.

THE ACTION PLAN

Once the assessment group has gathered the data and established priorities, a plan for action must be determined. This involves creating an **action plan** with concrete **action steps** (individual components of an action plan), a time line, and individuals responsible for the steps. *Healthy People* provides a good starting point from which to direct the action plan.

Objectives should have specific, measurable targets. We will use *Healthy People 2010* goal 15 and the data collected by a community needs assessment group in Northwest Indiana as an example. Remember, the process presented here is of major importance in achieving the goal of a healthy community. Also, this process may be used to address all of the *Healthy People 2010* goals.

Analysis of Table 7-2 reveals that, of the 39 *Healthy People 2010* objectives, the group was able to attain data on 13 objectives. The group must now assess these 13 objectives and determine which ones should be addressed for action.

For purposes of demonstration, we have selected objectives 19 and 23 for our action plan. These are: "increase use of safety belts" and "increase use of helmets by bicyclists." The group selected these two due to their impact on the youth in the community. The theory advanced was that if young citizens could be educated as to the importance of safety equipment while riding in automobiles and on bicycles, this would transfer to their adult lives and, therefore, to their children.

Figure 7-2 ▪ Checklist for Proposals

Proposal Abstract Checklist

Title: _____

Date Received: _____   Date Reviewed: _____

Areas	Not Included 0	Mini- mal 1	Suffi- cient 2	Thorough/ Outstanding 3
1. Explanation of how it furthers community goals				
2. Identification of target population				
3. Identification of health and well-being needs addressed				
4. Statement of purpose				
5. Identification of outcome(s)				
6. Project narrative				
7. Identification of region to benefit or participate				
8. Explanation of cross-disciplinary nature of project				
9. Identification of student engagement or service-learning				
10. Timeline				
11. Budget				
12. Identification of external funding sources				
13. Definition of health and well-being that is holistic and cross-disciplinary				
14. Addresses issue(s) of the community				
15. Sustainability				

Comments: Total Score:

TABLE 7-2 Example Needs Assessment: Reduce Injuries, Disabilities, and Deaths Due to Unintentional Injuries and Violence (*Healthy People 2010* [Conference Edition in Volume I] Washington, DC)

HP 2010	TARGET	DATA ASSESSED	NEED	RECOMMENDATIONS
1. Reduce hospitalization for nonfatal head injuries	To 54 hospitalizations / 100,000 population	No data available regarding head and spinal cord injuries per hospital, for the county or the State.	?	
2. Reduce hospitalization for nonfatal spinal cord injuries	To 2.6 hospitalizations / 100,000 population	No data available regarding head and spinal cord injuries per hospital, for the county or the State.	?	
3. Reduce firearm-related deaths	To 4.9 deaths / 100,000 population	The rates of homicide per 100,000 population for the state of Indiana for the year 1998 are: 7.7 (Bureau of Crime, 2000).	X	
4. Reduce the proportion of persons living in homes with firearms that are loaded and unlocked	To 16%	No data available regarding head and spinal cord injuries per hospital, for the county or the State.	?	
5. Reduce nonfatal firearm-related injuries	To 10.9 injuries / 100,000 population	In 1997, there were five deaths from firearms injuries in Lake county; no deaths from firearms injuries in LaPorte, and no deaths from firearms injuries in Porter counties (Data and Statistics, 1998).	X	
6. Extend State-level child fatality review of deaths due to external causes for children ≤ 14 years	Developmental	No data available.	?	

continues

TABLE 7-2   Example Needs Assessment: Reduce Injuries, Disabilities, and Deaths Due to Unintentional Injuries and Violence (*Healthy People 2010* [Conference Edition in Volume I] Washington, DC) *continued*

HP 2010	TARGET	DATA ASSESSED	NEED	RECOMMENDATIONS
7. Reduce nonfatal poisonings	To 292 nonfatal poisonings / 100,000 population	No data available.	?	
8. Reduce deaths caused by poisonings	To 1.8 deaths / 100,000 population	In Lake county for the year 1997, total age-adjusted death rate from injury and poisoning was 67.67; In LaPorte county for the year 1997, total age-adjusted death rate from injuries and poisonings was 60.53; In Porter county for the year 1997, total age-adjusted death rate from injuries and poisonings was 43.55. (Indiana Hospital, 1996–1997).	X	
9. Reduce deaths caused by suffocation	To 2.9 deaths / 100,000 population	No data available.	?	
10. Increase the number of States and the District of Columbia with state-wide emergency department surveillance systems that collect data on external causes of injury	States and the District of Columbia	Data collected on external causes of injury and reported annually through the annual Indiana Hospital Association.		

Objective	Target	Data	Status
11. Increase the number of States and the District of Columbia that collect data on external causes of injury through hospital discharge data systems	All States and the District of Columbia	Data collected on external causes of injury and reported annually through the annual Indiana Hospital Association.	
12. Reduce hospital emergency department visits caused by injuries	To 112 hospital emergency department visits / 1,000 population	No data available.	?
13. Reduce deaths caused by unintentional injuries	To 20.8 deaths / 100,000 population	In Lake county for the year 1997, total age-adjusted death rate from unintentional injuries and falls was 28.06; death rate from intentional injuries and adverse effects was 39.38; death rate from suicide was 8.23; death rate from homicide was 31.15 (Indiana Hospital, 1996–1997).	X
14. Reduce nonfatal unintentional injuries	Developmental		
15. Reduce deaths caused by motor vehicle crashes	To 9.0 deaths / 100,000 population for 15–15a and I deaths / 100 million vehicle miles traveled (VMT) for	In Lake county for the year 1997, total age-adjusted death rate from motor vehicle accidents was 12.72 (Indiana Hospital, 1996–1997).	X

continues

TABLE 7-2 Example Needs Assessment: Reduce Injuries, Disabilities, and Deaths Due to Unintentional Injuries and Violence (*Healthy People 2010* [Conference Edition in Volume I] Washington, DC) *continued*

HP 2010	TARGET	DATA ASSESSED	NEED	RECOMMENDATIONS
	15–15b (See HP2010 Volume I, p. 15–26 & 15–27)			
16. Reduce pedestrian deaths on public roads	To 1 pedestrian death / 100,000 population	No data available.	?	
17. Reduce nonfatal injuries caused by motor vehicle crashes	To 1,000 nonfatal injuries / 100,000 population	No data available.	?	
18. Reduce nonfatal pedestrian injuries on public roads	To 21 nonfatal injuries / 100,000 population	No data available.	?	
19. Increase use of safety belts	To 92%	In 1999, 16.4% of all adolescents nationwide never or rarely wore a seat belt (Youth Risk Behavior Survey, 1999).	X	
20. Increase use of child restraints	To 100%	No data available.	?	
21. Increase the proportion of motorcyclists using helmets	To 79%	In 1997 in Indiana, of a total of 62 motorcycle rider deaths, nine were helmeted and 49 (79.03%) were **unhelmeted** (National Highway Traffic Safety, 2000).	X	

22. Increase the number of States and the District of Columbia that have adopted a graduated driver licensing model law	To all States and the District of Columbia	No data readily available on plans to do so.	?
23. Increase use of helmets by bicyclists	Developmental	In 1999, 85.3% of adolescents nationwide **never** or rarely wore a bicycle helmet for students who rode bicycles (Youth Risk Behavior Survey, 1999).	X
24. Increase the number of States and the District of Columbia with laws requiring bicycle helmets for bicycle riders	All States and the District of Columbia	No data readily available.	?
25. Reduce residential fire deaths	To 0.6 deaths/ 100,000 population	No data available.	?
26. Increase functioning residential smoke alarms	To 100% for total population living in residences with smoke alarms on every floor, and residences with a functioning smoke alarm on every floor	No data available.	?

continues

TABLE 7-2 Example Needs Assessment: Reduce Injuries, Disabilities, and Deaths Due to Unintentional Injuries and Violence (*Healthy People 2010* [Conference Edition in Volume I] Washington, DC) *continued*

HP 2010	TARGET	DATA ASSESSED	NEED	RECOMMENDATIONS
27. Reduce deaths from falls	To 2.3 deaths / 100,000 population	In Lake county for the year 1997, total age-adjusted death rate from from unintentional injuries and falls was 28.06 (Indiana Hospital, 1996–1997).	X	
28. Reduce hip fractures among older adults	Rate / 100,000: To 491.0 for females > 65 years & 450.5 for males > 65 years	No data available.	?	
29. Reduce drownings	To 0.9 drownings / 100,000 population	In 1997, there were four drownings reported in Lake county, one drowning in LaPorte, and one drowning in Porter county (Data and Statistics, 1998).	?	
30. Reduce hospital emergency department visits for nonfatal dog bite injuries	To 114 hospital emergency department visits / 100,000 population	No data available.	?	
31. Increase the proportion of public and private schools that require use of appropriate head, face, eye, and mouth protection for students participa-	Developmental			

...ting in school-sponsored physical activities

Objective	Target	Finding	
32. Reduce homicide	To 3.2 homicides / 100,000 population	In Gary, the homicide-to-population ratio has steadily increased from 61 homicides for a population of 143,106 in 1985 to 98 homicides for a population of 116,481 in 1997 (Bureau of Crime, 2000).	X
33. Reduce maltreatment and maltreatment fatalities of children	Reduce maltreatment of children to 11.1 / 1,000 children < 18 years; Reduce child maltreatment fatalities to 1.5 / 100,000 children < 18 years	No data available.	?
34. Reduce the rate of physical assault by current or former intimate partners	To 3.6 physical assaults / 1,000 persons ≥ 12 years	In 1995, 8.4% of Gary adults, and 3.5% of Lake County adults were victims of domestic violence in the past five years (PRC Community Health Assessment, 1996).	?
35. Reduce the annual rate of rape or attempted rape	To 0.7 rapes or attempted rapes / 1,000 persons	In 1996, 1,992 rapes were reported in Indiana and resulted in 178 arrests (Office of Women's Health, 2000).	X
36. Reduce sexual assault other than rape	To 0.2 sexual assaults other than rape / 1,000 persons ≥ 12 years	No data available.	?

continues

TABLE 7-2 Example Needs Assessment: Reduce Injuries, Disabilities, and Deaths Due to Unintentional Injuries and Violence (*Healthy People 2010* [Conference Edition in Volume I] Washington, DC) *continued*

HP 2010	TARGET	DATA ASSESSED	NEED	RECOMMENDATIONS
37. Reduce physical assaults	To 25.5 physical assaults / 1,000 persons > 12 years	No data available for children > 12 years.	?	
38. Reduce physical fighting among adolescents	To 33.3%	In 1999, 5.2% of adolescents nationwide felt too unsafe to go to school at least one time in the last 30 day period; 35.7% were involved in a physical fight at least once in a 12 month period; and 14.2% were involved in a fight on school property at least once in a 12 month period (Youth Risk Behavior Survey, 1999).	X	
39. Reduce weapon carrying by adolescents on school property	To 6%	In 1999, 5.2% of adolescents nationwide felt too unsafe to go to school at least one time in the last 30 day period; 7.7% were threatened or injured with a weapon on school property at least once in a 12 month period; 4.9% had carried a gun on at least one occasion in a 30 day period; 6.9% carried a weapon on school property at least once in a 30 day period (Youth Risk Behavior Survey, 1999).	X	

STATEMENT OF COMMUNITY OBJECTIVES

At this point, we need to state specifically what we wish to achieve. Our community health objectives need to have specific targets. Ours may be stated as "Decrease the proportion of school age children who never or rarely use seat belts while riding in automobiles." Target: 8 percent by 2010. Baseline: 16 percent of all adolescents nationwide never or rarely wore a seat belt. Additionally, we believe that safety in automobiles may be improved by early use of safety equipment. Our second objective may be stated as "Increase the use of helmets while riding bicycles." Target: 50 percent by 2010. Baseline: 85 percent of adolescents never or rarely wore a bicycle helmet.

The target is a measurable outcome that we want to achieve within a certain time frame. Each objective should be measurable, wherever possible. How we will measure our targets should be determined early on so that we can properly follow our progress. Be realistic when setting targets. A target of 100 percent helmet wearers would be very admirable, but highly unlikely. Setting unrealistic targets can be very demoralizing and may jeopardize the success of a community health coalition.

ACTION STEPS

What concrete actions will we take to accomplish our targets? Should we offer safety programs at the local schools? Is it possible to obtain funding for free bicycle helmet giveaways? Should we contact auto dealers for support on seat belt use education? Is there funding for a reward system that the local police or neighborhood watch groups could administer when they observe helmet users? Is there an organization in the community that could spearhead a public relations campaign? How will we collect data on the results? Who will provide reports to whom? When do we need reports?

A good deal of time will be spent identifying and selecting the action steps needed to reach our desired targets. The action steps need to be very specific, with persons responsible and time frames identified. Assigning specific individuals to action steps will help accomplish the objectives, as will realistic time frames. Recall that we have several years to achieve our objectives.

IMPLEMENTING THE ACTION PLAN

Implement the plan of the coalition by taking concrete actions that will make a difference. A prepared list of action steps provides an excellent starting point to assign coalition members responsibility for specific tasks, according to an agreed-upon time frame. The team as a group needs to charge individuals formally with the tasks while the individuals must formally accept the responsibility of seeing the task through to fruition. Our coalition may or may not have community leaders who can help accomplish the action steps. Implementation is assisted if the leaders are already on board. If not, enlisting their support and help may be an action step in and of itself.

TRACKING PROGRESS

Another element of an action plan is routine tracking of events. Monthly or quarterly reports should be required as part of a monitoring system to help the team follow the progress of the action plan. Patience is a requisite quality of the coalition team. Organizing and involving people in community action plans take time, sometimes more than expected or merited for the action at hand. Good things come to those who wait, but not to those who fail to plan.

 KEY POINTS

Analysis can take many forms and shapes, requiring the application of a variety of research tools and techniques.

Action planning must be included in analysis without which the four steps of the Ontario Needs Impact Based Model would be practically useless. It is not enough to know, if there is no plan to do.

◆ Research, tools, and techniques include: the scientific method, the survey method, the Delphi method, SPSS, QSR NVivo, and descriptive statistics.

◆ Grant proposals may be necessary to attain funding to reach the objective of a healthy community.

◆ The steps in an action plan include statement of community objective(s), action steps, implementation, and tracking progress.

 REFERENCES

Anderson, E., & McFarlane, J. (2000). *Community as partner: Theory and practice in nursing.* (3rd ed.) New York: Lippincott/Williams & Wilkins.

Blair, J., Rock, T., Rotarius, T., Fottler, M., et al, (1996). The problematic fit of diagnosis and strategy for medical group stakeholders—including IDS/Ns. *Health Care Management Review, 21,* 7–23.

Dalkey, N., & Helmer, O. (1963, April). An experimental application of the Delphi method to the uses of experts, *Management Science, 9,* 458–67.

Fox, N., & Roberts, C. (1999). GPs in cyberspace: The sociology of a "virtual community." *Sociological Review, 47,* 643–669.

Leedy, P. (1980). *Practical research* (2nd ed.) New York: Macmillan.

Nardi, D., Sutherland, T., Tippy, F., & Strupeck, D. (2000). *Needs assessment of the health and wellbeing of Northwest Indiana.* Indiana University Northwest, Shared Vision Research and Service Task Forces. Unpublished manuscript.

National Geographic Society. (2000). *Survey 2000* [online]. Available: survey2000.nationalgeographic.com.

Richards, L. (1999). Data alive! The thinking behind NVivo. *Qualitative Health Research, 9* (3).

Rodeghier, M. (1966). *Surveys with confidence: A Practical guide to survey research using SPSS.* Chicago: SPSS, Inc.

Rosenstock, L., Olenec, C., & Wagner, G. (1998). The National Occupational Research Agenda: A model of broad stakeholder input into priority setting. *American Journal of Public Health, 88,* 353–356.

Rowe, G., & Wright, G. (1999). The Delphi technique as a forecasting tool: Issues and analysis. *International Journal of Forecasting, 15,* 353–375.

Rueschhoff, N., & Strupeck, D. (1998). Equity returns: Local GAAP versus U.S. GAAP for foreign issuers from developing countries, *International Journal of Accounting, 33* (3), 377–389.

Schmidt, R. C. 1997. Managing Delphi surveys using nonparametric statistical techniques. *Decision Sciences, 28* (3), 763–774.

Schutt, R. (2001). *Investigating the social world* (3rd ed.). Thousand Oaks, CA: Pine Forge Press.

Tornquist, E. (1986). *From proposal to publication: An informal guide to writing about nursing research.* Menlo Park, CA: Addison Wesley.

U.S. Department of Health and Human Services. (2001). *Healthy people in healthy communities: A community planning guide using Healthy People 2010.* Washington, DC: U.S. Government Printing Office.

RESOURCES FOR DATA GATHERING AND COMPARISON

Martin A. Kremer

 LEARNING OBJECTIVES

At the conclusion of this chapter, the reader will be able to:

- ◆ Locate Internet resources suitable for use in developing a health and wellness assessment.
- ◆ Describe the differences between reliable and suspect Internet sources.
- ◆ Choose a search engine that will match his or her own investigative needs.

KEY TERMS

Compressed file or archive	Search engine
Database	Self-extracting archive
Download	Spreadsheet
HTML	Table
Internet	Uniform resource locator (URL)
Internet service provider (ISP)	Web page and web site
Node	World Wide Web

This chapter examines resources available to health care and human services providers for use in identifying leading health indicators and national, regional, and local benchmarks. It focuses on freely accessible Internet resources, and includes some primary data sources, principally as examples of the kinds of sources available at the time of this writing. Resources are organized into categories alphabetically so that they can be more directly related to the task of creating a health needs assessment under *Healthy People 2010* guidelines.

RESEARCH THEN AND NOW, THE OBVIOUS

As recently as 15 years ago, researchers looking for existing data were limited to gathering data by poring over printed indexes of published materials and then retrieving or requesting the material from a library. Often, a library would not have the requested material among its holdings. There ensued the potentially lengthy process of requesting the material from another library, and the fevered reading of the material in order to return it by the due date (which was never far enough in the future for the researcher's liking). Even when the researcher's primary library held the materials needed, the researcher faced difficulty. Periodicals and major references are seldom permitted to leave a library. The resulting photocopying costs did nothing to erase the image of the impoverished academic researcher.

A researcher today can work anywhere there is a computer with a modem and a telephone connection. The **Internet** is a global network of computers. Originally created by the U.S. Department of Defense (DOD) to connect universities working on DOD projects, the Internet has grown to encompass every kind of human activity. At first, the Internet was a text-only, command-line medium that worked based on command words typed into the computer. The first step to using the Internet was learning dozens of commands and the specific ways they were to be typed. The development of the World Wide Web has changed the character of the Internet, making it available and easy to use for anyone with a computer and an Internet connection. The **World Wide Web** provides a way of combining multiple files from the Internet into a single presentation via a program known as a browser, which can combine text, pictures, and even sounds into a single **web page.** A collection of these pages on a single computer is known as a **web site.** Most navigation through web sites is done by clicking on words or pictures that are associated with **Uniform Resource Locators (URLs).** A URL is a string of characters that uniquely identifies a file on a computer somewhere on the Internet.

Working at home or in the office with a computer and a connection to the Internet, a researcher today has access to information far wider in scope and much more easily than a print-only counterpart. Internet connections are not simply a phone line, but a service you must purchase through an **Internet service provider (ISP).** There are many local ISPs and a number of large national ISPs, such as America On Line. (Shopping for an ISP is beyond the scope of this book and will not be addressed here.)

Once connected to the Internet, a researcher can visit a web site such as Yahoo!, type in a few words to identify the information she is interested in, and have immediate access to other web sites around the world that in one way or another meet her search criteria. The information accessed in this way can be read on-screen, printed out (usually) at the researcher's own printer, perhaps **downloaded,** cut and pasted into a word processing document or spreadsheet, or, in the worst of all possible situations, copied by hand onto a 3 x 5 note card for later transcription.

... AND THE NOT SO OBVIOUS

There is, however, a dark side to Internet research. On the one hand, you can find anything on the Internet. On the other hand, you can find *any*thing on the Internet. When journals and books were the primary source of information for researchers, the task was to find information. When using the Internet, the task is to find *good* information.

When paper and ink were the only ways to publish information, a system of checks and balances grew that tended to encourage honesty among writers, researchers, editors, and publishers. The reason was primarily economic. Publishers were unwilling to spend the money to print articles or books that could damage their reputation or fail in the marketplace because of faulty research. Editors were unwilling to risk their jobs by printing articles or books that would cost the publisher money. The entire infrastructure of blind review developed to help the publisher avoid printing flawed, bad, or fraudulent research. The editor knows who the author is and who the reviewers are, but the author does not know who reviews her work and the reviewer does not know whose work he is reviewing. This is still the process followed by book and journal publishers who value their reputations, and it permits us to accept without doubt that an article in, say, the *Journal of the American Medical Association* meets specific standards of research practice and reporting.

These checks and balances, however, do not necessarily apply to research published on the Internet. The explosive growth of the Internet over the past few years has led to a state in which everyone can, and seemingly almost everyone does, have a web site. Anything and everything exists on the Internet. And while responsible organizations follow the same standards and practices for electronic as well as print media, not every organization or individual with a web site feels the need to hold to such stringent standards. Individual web site owners can and do publish whatever they please. Organizations with more agenda than integrity do the same, but with the added patina of respectability that comes with a .org or .edu web site name. The responsibility for discriminating between valid and invalid data, valuable and worthless information, truth and falsehood falls directly on the researcher using the Internet. The researcher therefore would be well advised to heed the ancient Latin maxim, *caveat emptor.* In a later section, we'll look at ways to reduce the chances of using flawed data.

FINDING WHAT YOU WANT ON THE INTERNET

Finding printed material, especially periodical articles, often requires access to a published index such as the Cumulative Index to Nursing and Allied Health (CINAHL) or ERIC. These indexes are now usually available as electronic **databases,** but are not normally open to public access. The researcher will usually need to access these electronic indexes from a college or university library terminal or establish a user ID in order to use them from a home computer. Using them from outside an academic environment frequently requires payment for the service.

The major advantage to these indexes is that they often permit direct access to full-text electronic copies of the indexed articles, which ultimately saves time. Older issues of indexed periodicals, however, may still be available only through printed indexes. In this case, the researcher must fall back on the skills developed during pre-electronic life, which are beyond the scope of this discussion.

Public Internet resources use programs called **search engines** to locate information. Search engines do not actually search the Internet for items that match a request. Instead, they search pre-built indexes. These indexes are built in a number of ways: some indexes are created through systematic browsing of web sites, capturing content information directly from the pages themselves, others by accepting category information provided on a questionnaire by the owner of the web page. The indexing used by search engines can lead to some odd results. It is not uncommon for a search to return no results. This is usually due to specifying search requirements too narrowly. Changing the requirements in a seemingly trivial way can result in the next search returning hundreds of thousands of matches.

The real trick to using a search engine is to find one whose indexing scheme matches your own—or, more accurately, one whose designer thinks as you do. A search engine is a computer program that queries a large database of index entries and returns the results to your browser. The organization of that database, especially the words chosen to build the index and the way that those words can be combined to identify matches, has a direct relationship to your level of comfort with the search engine. The best way to determine which search engine suits you is to test-drive as many as you can find.

Netscape Navigator and Microsoft Internet Explorer are the most popular browsers available today, and each has a 'Search' button on its Navigation Toolbar. Pressing the 'Search' button while connected to the Internet will display the search site provided by the company. These sites will permit you to select search engines such as Alta Vista, Ask Jeeves, Google, GoTo, LookSmart, Lycos, Northern Light, and Yahoo! Choose a search word or phrase that you feel distinguishes the information you want to retrieve and use it on each of the available search engines. The engines are likely to return a common subset of sites, but each will have sites that are extraneous to your needs. Occasionally, an engine will return exactly what you are looking for as its first result. Review the sites. Repeat this process several times, looking for something different each time. The engine that consistently brings back the most useful sites with the lowest number of unhelpful sites is a good bet for your primary search engine. But even after you have chosen the search engine that best suits you, remember to check back with other engines when your primary choice doesn't bring you what you need.

GRABBING THE DATA

Data exists in dozens of formats on the Internet. Some formats are more useful than others, and some require more work than others in order to get something useful. In addition, while some data is available as the data processing equivalent of a fully prepared seven-course meal, some is more like groceries. Sites like the Behavioral Risk Factor Surveillance System, a part of the Centers for Disease Control (http://www.cdc.gov/nccdphp/brfss/index.htm), contain a full range of information, from raw data, to discrete statistics, to reports on the data including statistical analysis of the raw data broken down by state. This raw data, however, is *a lot* of data. For one year of this questionnaire's raw data, the **compressed file** size is 19MB, and unless you are focusing on this particular question, probably not worth the hours of time it would take to download at phone-line speeds. In most cases, however, you will be looking for a smaller set of data. The analysis of the raw data is typically a much smaller file. Occasionally, you will be looking for a quotation to present your interpretation of the data succinctly. In this case, you may need only a few words or lines from the web site or a report.

To get a few lines from a web site, it is almost always possible to highlight and copy text, and sometimes even small- to medium-size data tables, directly from the web site. If the site resists this kind of copying, you can choose the 'View' menu option, typically the third item from the left, following 'File' and 'Edit'. From the menu that drops down, choose 'Source' (Internet Explorer) or 'Page Source' (Navigator). This will show you the native **HTML (HyperText Markup Language)** that is being interpreted and displayed as the web page. This can be copied and pasted into your document, but will require some cleanup since the HTML will include formatting commands that will need to be removed. HTML is the basic language of the World Wide Web, and provides instructions embedded in the text that tell your browser how to display the page.

Tables are gridlike formats for holding data. They appear very much like **spreadsheets,** with data organized into columns representing variables and rows representing cases. They often present a special difficulty when copied from a web page. They do not paste into other documents very well. In these cases it is usually best to copy the source as described above, but to paste the results into a program known as an HTML editor. There are dozens of free HTML editors available on the Internet. Just use your search engine to locate "Free HTML editor" entries and pick one from the results. Tables will always begin with the text '<table>' and end with '</table>'. These are HTML tags that tell the browser how to interpret the text that comes between them. Copy from the <table> tag to the </table>

tag, including the tags. Then paste the copied text into a web page document between the <body> and </body> tags. Save this file and then insert it into your word processing document using the 'Insert . . . file' menu options

Very often, the site designer will give you a very straightforward way to download a file. Simply click on a link on the page and if the file referenced by the link is not an HTML file, your browser will begin to download the file from the Internet. If your browser is configured to automatically open files downloaded in this way, you will soon be viewing the file in Word or Excel or WordPerfect or Adobe Acrobat Reader. But this is not always the best choice. It is usually better in the long run to choose the 'Save to disk' option, since in that case you will have greater control over where the file is saved and will be able to give the file a name that is reasonably descriptive of the contents. Some site designers will permit you to download **self-extracting archive** files that, after downloading, are executed as if they were programs, to extract the compressed files.

Some sites may offer you the option of ordering the data you need on diskette or CD-ROM. This will usually require the payment of a fee for copying and mailing, but is well worth the few dollars it will cost if you really need the data and cannot get a download to work.

Purchasers of this book have an additional resource available at the Delmar Learning web site. On the site dedicated to this book is a document containing skeleton tables for each of the *Healthy People 2010* goals. The objectives for each of the goals and the targets have already been filled in. The tables also have blank columns to identify data being collected, identify whether this is an observed need, and list recommendations to address the need.

SEPARATING THE WHEAT FROM THE CHAFF

Before the advent of the World Wide Web, the only available methods of publishing involved either submitting to editorial oversight or bearing the expense of publishing oneself. The Web has made the vanity press affordable to anyone who has the wherewithal to subscribe to an Internet service. Given the variable value of data that can be found on the Internet, how can a researcher ever be confident of the data she finds there? What constitutes due diligence in using data that comes without the imprimatur of a known publisher, or the names of an editorial review board who deemed the material worthy of publication? Winnowing through the massive volume of available information and finding something worthwhile can be a daunting task. But it need not be overwhelming. By following a few basic rules, researchers can feel confident that they are not going to regret using any particular source of information.

The U.S. government is a trustworthy source of raw data and statistical information. Government web sites will always have web address that begin www.something.gov/ Sites owned by reputable organizations like the American Diabetes Association or the American Cancer Society are also trustworthy and have long-term data collection and reporting available. These sites carry the.org designation. Other sites that can usually be trusted are those ending in.edu. These represent educational institutions. There is, however, potential danger lurking in these sites. In order to qualify for a.org address, all that need be shown is proof of nonprofit status. Thus some organizations can register as churches and request a.org web address. In the world of.edu addresses, universities and even some high schools afford their faculty and students space to publish a web site and these sites are not necessarily monitored for accurate content.

The most effective way to ensure that an article or data source on the web is trustworthy is to cross-check the source. This involves extra work, but is worth the effort if it saves you from quoting the lunatic fringe.

1. Look for other sources that cite the source or author in question. Finding such citations in journals of known respectability is a good indication that the source can be trusted. Be aware, however, that not finding a citation of the source does not mean the source is untrustworthy. Researchers and authors often spend several years writing and publishing before they reach the point where they are included in the references of other authors.

2. Check the citations in the source in question. Serious researchers will have a preponderance of identifiable sources. A data source that cites only its own author may not have a wide enough knowledge base to be accepted without further checking.

3. An author who denigrates positions other than his own is violating one of the basic rules of research. Let the data speak. If the data disagrees with other researchers, the subject is open to debate but not personal attack.

4. Use your search engine to look for other works by the same author. Finding the author in print journals rather than Internet-only publications gives weight to the author's credentials.

IT WAS RIGHT HERE YESTERDAY!

Sooner or later, everyone comes face to face with the dreaded '404 Not Found' error, or worse yet, the 'cannot find server' error. These errors can cause responses ranging from anger and frustration all the way to sheer panic, depending upon how desperately you need the information on the page that cannot be located. The 404 error can result from a wide range of circumstances, but can often be resolved by following a few simple steps.

1. If you typed in the URL, try typing it again. Perhaps you misspelled something.

2. If you selected the address from your 'favorites' list, try removing the right-hand parts of the address one **node** at a time. In other words, start by removing the '/something.html' portion of the name and pressing the 'Enter' key. This will cause the browser to look for anything in the lowest level directory still showing in the address box. Continue in this way, removing everything from the rightmost slash to the end of the line and then pressing 'Enter' until, with luck, you get something other than a 404 error. If you get a web page, wonderful. If you get a 'Index of' page with just a text list, try clicking on one of the .htm or .html names. From this point, you may be able to navigate to your information from the page that is then displayed.

3. If you get all the way down to 'www.something.something' and still cannot find your web site, it is still not time to panic. Some kinds of system maintenance require the site be off-line, and the site may be available again after an hour or so. If you still have no luck, go back to your favorite search engine and begin searching for the content you need. If this doesn't work on the day you first try it, wait a day or two and try again. Search indexes are not updated immediately. If a site has changed its name, it will take a little time for the indexes to be brought up to date.

4. The worst-case scenario is that the site you are looking for no longer exists anywhere. If this is the case, it may be wise to go back and review the "Separating the Wheat from the Chaff" section above. Sites that disappear overnight may signal any number of things. An organization may have gone out of business, an individual may have switched service providers, or the web site owner may have restructured its web facility. However, organizations providing high-quality content will not often disappear entirely.

INTERNET RESOURCES

The following resources were available as cited at the time of this writing. Keep in mind that the caveat regarding disappearing web sites can apply to these as well.

General Resources

◆ Heartland Center. (2000).
Available: http://www.theteimsonline.com/org/heartland/
newcensus.html

◆ National Academies of Sciences, (2000).
Available: http://www.nationalacademies.org/

◆ O'Brien, R. (1998). An overview of the methodological approach of
action research. Action research methodology.
Available: http://www.web.net/~robrien/papers/arfinal.html

◆ Ottawa Charter for Health Promotion. (1986). Geneva: WHO.
Available: http://www.helsetilsynet.no/trykksak/fremmdok/
glossary.html

◆ U.S. Census Bureau: U.S. Department of Commerce.
Available: http://www.census.gov/

Healthy People 2010

◆ Public Health Foundation *Healthy People 2010* Tool Library.
Available: http://www.phf.org/HPtools/state.html

◆ Centers for Disease Control. (2000). DATA 2010: The Healthy
People Database.
Available: http://wonder.cdc.gov/nios.shtml

Goal 1. Access to Quality Health Services

◆ Heale, J. & Abernathy, T. (1996). *Community health planning:
Determining the needs of the community.*
Available: http://cwhweb.mdmaster.ca/planning/itch96.html

Goal 2. Arthritis, Osteoporosis, and Chronic Back Conditions

◆ The Arthritis Foundation research page.
Available: http://www.arthritis.org/research/default.asp

◆ National Institutes of Health Osteoporosis and Related Bone
Diseases National Resource Center.
Available: http://www.osteo.org/

Goal 3. Cancer

◆ American Cancer Society.
Available: http://www.cancer.org/

Goal 4. Chronic Kidney Disease

♦ National Institute of Diabetes and Digestive and Kidney Diseases.
Available: http://www.niddk.nih.gov/

♦ Medscape Urology.
Available: http://urology.medscape.com/home/topics/urology/
urology.html

Goal 5. Diabetes

♦ American Diabetic Association. (2000). *Diabetes: Indiana's health
problem.*
Available: http://www.diabetes.org

Goal 6. Disability and Secondary Conditions

♦ U.S. Census Bureau.
Available: http://www.census.gov/hhes/www/disable/dissipp.html

Goal 7. Educational and Community-Based Programs

♦ Community Health Status Indicators Project. (2000). Washington,
DC. U.S. Department of Health and Human Services.
Available: http://www.communityhealth.hrsa.gov/

Goal 8. Environmental Health

♦ Long-range Air Transport of Dioxin from North American Sources
to Ecologically Vulnerable Receptors in Nunavut, Arctic Canada.
Final Report to the North American Commission for Environmental
Cooperation. (2000, September).
Available: http://www.cec.org/programs_projects/pollutants_health/
develop_tools/dioxins/dioxexec.pdf

♦ Ozone Season Report, IDEM, Office of Air Management. (2000,
January).
Available: http:///www.state.in.us/idem/oam/standard/nwind/
index.html

♦ Pew Environmental Health Commission. (2000). Attack asthma:
Why America needs a public health defense system to battle envi-
ronmental threats.
Available: http://pewenvirohealth.jhsph.edu/html/splash/text.html

♦ U.S. Air Quality Nonattainment Areas. (2000).
Available: http://www.epa.gov/airs/nonattn.html

♦ U.S. Environmental Protection Agency. (1999). Facts about wetlands.
Available: www.epa.gov/owow/wetlands/facts/fact5.html

◆   U.S. Environmental Protection Agency. (1998). Toxic release
    inventory.
    Available: http://www.epa.gov/opptintrl/tri/states.html

◆   U.S. Environmental Protection Agency.
    Available: http:///www.epa.gov/

Goal 9. Family Planning

◆   Population Council.
    Available: http://www.popcouncil.org/sfp/default.asp

Goal 10. Food Safety

◆   *Fish Consumption Advisory.* (2000).
    Available: http://www.state.in.us./isdh/dataandstats/fish/fish_2000/
    group_5_waterways.html

Goal 11. Health Communication

◆   National Center for Chronic Disease Prevention & Health
    Promotion. (2000). Behavioral Risk Factor Surveillance System.
    BRFFS prevalence data.
    Available: http://www2.cdc.gov/nccdphp/brffs/index.asp

◆   National Association for Public Health Statistics and Information
    Systems. (2000).
    Available: http://38.180.50.49/Main/home.html

Goal 12. Heart Disease and Stroke

◆   American Heart Association.
    Available: http://www.americanheart.org/

Goal 13. HIV

◆   Body Health Resources Corporation AIDS information web site.
    Available: www.thebody.com

Goal 14. Immunization and Infectious Diseases

◆   Data and Statistics. (1998). Epidemiology Resource Center (ERC).
    Available: www.state.in.us/isdh/

◆   World Surveillance Report—Selected Data Highlights. (1996).
    Selected data highlights: Pneumoconiosis mortality.
    Available: http://www.cdc.gov/niosh/w7_high.html

Goal 15. Injury and Violence Prevention

◆   Bureau of Crime & Justice Electronic Data Abstracts. (2000). Crime
    & Justice Electronic Data Abstracts.
    Available: http://ww.ojp.usdoj.gov/bjs/dtdata.html

- Youth Behavior Risk Survey (YRBS). 1991, 1993, 1995, 1997, 1999. (2000). *Youth risk behavior trends.*
  Available: http://www.cdc.gov/nccdphp/dash/yrbs/trend.html

- MADD Statistics 1999 Fatalities by State. (1999).
  Available: http://www.madd.org/stats99_fataliities_by_state.shtml

- National Center for Injury Prevention and Control. (2000).
  Available: http://webappp.cdc.gov/cgi-bin/broker.exe?

- National Highway Traffic Safety Administration. (1996). State of Indiana Toll of Mortor Vehicle Crashes, 1996.
  Available: http://www.nhtsa.dot.gov/people/ncsa/stateinfo/ indiana.html

- Office of Women's Health. (2000). Violence against women.
  Available: http://www.state.in.us/isdh/programs/owh/ violence.html

Goal 16. Maternal, Infant, and Child Health

- Brody, T., King, P. & LeBlang, J. (1999). *County and zip code blood-lead data for children under six years of age testing above ten micrograms per deciliter in Region 5 states.* Chicago, IL: U.S. Environmental Protection Agency.
  Available: http:///www.epa.gov/reg5foia/reach/documents/ blood_lead_data.pdf

- Centers for Disease Control and Prevention Reproductive Health Information Source. (2000). Pregnancy risk assessment monitoring system.
  Available: http://www.cdc.gov/nccdphp/drh/srv_prams.html

- National Campaign to Prevent Teen Pregnancy. (1999). *Fact sheet: Teen pregnancy and childrearing in Indiana.*
  Available: http://www.teenpregnancy.org/usa/in.html

Goal 17. Medical Product Safety

- U.S. Food and Drug Administration. (2000). MedWatch: The FDA Medical Products Reporting Program.
  Available: http://www.fda.gov/medwatch/

- U.S. Food and Drug Administration—Center for Devices and Radiological Health. (2000).Final Report of a Study to Evaluate the Feasibility and Effectiveness of a Sentinel Reporting System for Adverse Event Reporting of Medical Device Use in User Facilities, June 16, 1999.

Available: http://www.fda.gov/cdrh/postsurv/ medsunappendixa.html

◆ U.S. Food and Drug Administration—Center for Drug Evaluation and Research. (2000). AERS—Adverse Event Reporting System. Available: http://www.fda.gov/cder/aers/index.html

Goal 18. Mental Health and Mental Disorders

◆ *Mental health: A report of the Surgeon General.* (1999). Available: http://www.surgeongeneral.gov/library/mentalhealth/ home.html

Goal 19. Nutrition and Overweight

◆ National Center for Chronic Disease Prevention and Health Promotion. Available: http://www.cdc.gov/nccdphp/dnpa/sitemap.html.

Goal 20. Occupational Safety and Health

◆ Bureau of Labor Statistics, U.S. Department of Labor, Survey of Occupational Injuries and Illnesses. (1998). Table 6. Available: http://stats.bls.gov/news.release/cfoi.t05.html

◆ National Institute for Occupational, Safety and Health. (1994). Silicosis deaths among young adults: United States 1968–1994. Available: www.epo.cdc.gov

◆ Safety and Health Statistics. (1999). *Table 5: fatal occupational injuries by State and event or exposure, 1999.* Available: http://stats.bls.gov/news.release/cfor.t05.html

Goal 21. Oral Health

◆ Association of State and Territorial Dental Directors. (2000). *Oral health access & disparities.* Available: http://www.astd.org/surgeon.html

Goal 22. Physical Activity and Fitness

◆ President's Council on Physical Fitness and Sports. Available: http://www.fitness.gov/activity/activity.html

◆ National Center for Chronic Disease Prevention and Health Promotion. Available: http://www.cdc.gov/nccdphp/dnpa/ physicalactivity.html

Goal 23. Public Health Infrastructure

◆ Public Health Practice Program Office. Available: http://www.phppo.cdc.gov/

Goal 24. Respiratory Diseases

◆ American Lung Association.
Available: http://www.lungusa.org/

Goal 25. Sexually Transmitted Diseases

◆ Dictionary of demographic and reproductive health terminology.
(1999). In *United Nations Population Information Network
(POPIN)*.
Available: http://www.popin.org/~unpopterms/default.html

Goal 26. Substance Abuse

◆ Changing the conversation: A national plan to improve substance
abuse. Chicago, IL. Public hearing. (1999).
Available: www.NaTxPlan.org/Chicago_Hearing.html

◆ CNN Health Story Page. (2000). *Genital herpes infection rate on the
rise*.
Available: http://www.cnn.com/HEALTH/9710/15/herpes/increase/

◆ National Household Survey on Drug Abuse. (1998).
Available: http://www.samhsa.gov/OAS/p0000016.html

Goal 27. Tobacco Use

◆ CDC Tobacco Information-State & National Tobacco Control
Highlights—Indiana. (2000).
Available: http://www.cdc.gov/tobacco/statehi/htmltext/in_sh.html

◆ American Cancer Society.
Available: http://www.cancer.org/

◆ American Lung Association.
Available: http://www.lungusa.org/

Goal 28. Vision and Hearing

◆ Better Hearing Institute. (2000). *Facts about hearing disorders*.
Available: http://www.betterhearing.org/demograp.html

◆ American Academy of audiology. (2000). *Status of hearing screening in each state*.
Available: http://www.infanthearing.org/statsu/unhsstate.html

GLOSSARY

Action Plan is a step-by-step, structured plan tailored to achieve a community's objectives.

Action Research is participatory research incorporating community service, addressing real problems in the real-world contexts of its communities. Its purpose is to effect societal change.

Action Steps are the individual components of an action plan.

Acute Disease is a disease having a sudden onset.

Analysis is the study and examination of data.

Benchmarks are targets for performance, or outcomes that indicate a goal has been reached.

Cardiovascular refers to the heart and its structures and related blood vessels. The heart is composed of cardiac muscle and blood vessels to which it is connected. The vessels are called veins and arteries and are the vehicles through which the blood is carried to other organs as it is pumped by the heart.

Carrying Capacity refers to the rate of use at which resources can be renewed or restored.

Catchment Area is a geographical region with distinct boundaries, encompassing anywhere from 75,000 to 200,000 residents, in which a community mental health center is designated to provide mental health services for the residents.

Chronic Disease is slow in onset and lifelong in consequences. A chronic disease is an illness that cannot be cured but can be controlled. A person may have many chronic diseases and yet feel relatively healthy. Also, the treatment may be extensive and can be catastrophic in cost due to recurrent ex-

acerbations or recurrence of the disease process. When a client with a chronic disease becomes ill with an involvement of that particular disease process, that client is usually sicker than one who is healthy. Therefore, because the client with a chronic disease is already sick or debilitated because of the preexisting condition, but yet stable with that condition, it takes longer for the person to get better when a recurrence of that disease process occurs.

Coalition is a group of individuals from an organization, neighborhood, or other constituency who are partnering, sharing resources, and cooperating in a specific work or a task in order to achieve the same goal. Coalitions are a necessary component of any community health and wellness assessment, since all community health endeavors should be conducted in partnership with the community.

Community refers to groups composed of individuals, families, organizations, or businesses that share a common language, values, history, or common purpose.

Community Intervention refers to a planned change initiative that is based on one or more community-based indicators.

Community Mental Health Centers are service centers within a specified community designation created through the joint efforts of the federal and state government to provide services to intervene with early and intensive treatment for those with mental illness and to promote mental health.

Community Objectives, are the identified determinants of health, as identified by *Healthy People 2010,* for a specific population.

Community Status Reports are hard copy and electronic vehicles that are used to describe and report community-based indicators.

Community Support System (CSS) is a model for community-based mental health services with multiple components that are primarily developed and implemented by an assigned community mental health center. Services include client identification and outreach, mental health treatment, health and dental care, crisis response services, protection and advocacy, rehabilitation, family and community support, peer support, income support, and entitlement and housing.

Comparative Needs are the identified determinants of health as identified by *Healthy People 2010* for a specific population, which are compared to the health behaviors outcome data for a specific population.

Compressed File or Archive is a file that has been modified by a program such as PKZip© to reduce its size. The smaller file takes up less disk drive space and can be transmitted over Internet or phone connections more quickly. The same program, or a compatible program, can then uncompress the file at its destination. These programs, with some advanced features and functions disabled, are available for free download from the Internet. See also **Self-Extracting Archive.**

Conceptual Framework is a linkage of concepts about a phenomenon to be studied that explains the relationships among the concepts. It provides a guideline for understanding what is known about the phenomenon under study and what needs to be known about it.

Continuous Improvement is associated with the Total Quality Management (TQM) movement, which is, in turn, associated with W. Edward Deming (1986) and Joseph Juran (1974). The term refers to the iterative use of data to improve work processes.

Culture refers to a pattern of values, beliefs and behaviors that a population or group demonstrates. This cultural pattern will influence how a target population views and values health and wellness, and how it accesses and uses health and wellness services.

Dashboard Indicators are a select set of indicators that speak to the health of a complex system.

Database is a file or group of files organized in such a way as to permit analysis of data by use of structured query language (SQL).

Deinstitutionalization was the movement of clients diagnosed with mental disorders from state mental hospitals and the shift in providing community-based mental health services within community settings (families, supervised nursing homes, and apartments).

Delphi Method is a research survey process that builds consensus as to expert opinions regarding relative issues.

Determinants of Health are critical influences, such as individual lifestyles, biologic makeup and behaviors, community physical, spiritual, and social environments, access to health care, and policies and health interventions that combine to shape and influence the health and wellness of individuals, families, and communities.

Developmental Goal is a goal that is established whenever there is a need to develop a baseline of information about the phenomenon under study.

Download is the process of copying a file from a central repository to another computer. As used here, it refers to copying from the Internet to a user's workstation.

Early Intervention is a coordinated system of services for infants and toddlers who have or are at risk for developmental disabilities, designed to prevent or minimize the disability to the degree possible.

Epidemiological Study is a type of action research that examines the distribution and determinants of health and wellness-related states for identified populations, and applies findings to the prevention, treatment, and control of health and health-related problems.

Expressed Needs related to health are the needs that are identified already by the users and providers of health care and community services in a community.

Felt Needs are any health indicators that people are aware of that are lacking or that they desire and do not have. A felt need may be shaped by a person's perceptions of the desirability of achieving a health indicator, or access to services.

Fetal Alcohol Syndrome (FAS) is a birth defect in infants of mothers who consumed alcohol during pregnancy. Effects include mental retardation, behavior and growth problems, structural abnormalities of the face and limbs, and other abnormalities. The degree of involvement is related to the amount of alcohol consumed and the duration and pregnancy stage in which it oc-

curred. No specific amount of alcohol is known to be a cause, hence abstinence during pregnancy is recommended.

Folic Acid is a B vitamin that is necessary for prevention of neural tube deficits such as spina bifida from developing in an embryo. The recommended daily allowance is 400 micrograms, with an additional 400 micrograms needed in pregnancy (Boyle & Zyla, 1996).

Full Employment means that the worker is employed full-time, or 40 hours per week, with customary benefits such as individual and family health insurance and vacation/illness pay.

Goals are broadly worded focus areas that provide direction for action and guides an assessment. *Healthy People*'s 28 goals, or focus areas, were derived from its two overarching goals to improve quality and length of life and eliminate heath disparities.

Health is defined using the World Health Organization (WHO) definition that describes it as a "state of complete physical, mental and social wellness and not merely the absence of disease or infirmity" (WHO, 2001, p.1) This broad definition of health emphasizes the importance of social factors such as socioeconomic status, education, safety, and the environment in the overall determination of the health of the community and the individual.

Healthy Community is a term used to describe any community that "embraces the belief that health is more than merely an absence of disease; a healthy community includes those elements that enable people to maintain a high quality of life and productivity" (Office of

Disease Prevention and Health Promotion, 2001, p. 1). The concept of the healthy community has been used as a conceptual foundation for community-based indicators initiatives.

Healthy People refers to a federal initiative that is based on two principles: (1) a belief that health is determined by a broad range of physical, environmental, social, economic, and behavioral factors; and (2) a commitment to the community-based amelioration of disparities in health outcomes. The *Healthy People* concept, which is closely related to the idea of the "healthy community," has been used as a conceptual foundation for community-based indicators initiatives.

HTML—Hyper Text Markup Language is the basic language in which web pages are written. It permits text to be interpreted by a browser to display a formatted page.

HTTP—Hyper Text Transaction Protocol is the underlying structure of web pages, and specifies the way that the text in files should be displayed on a computer screen.

Human Immunodeficiency Virus (HIV) is a virus that is the causative agent of the disease Auto Immune Deficiency Syndrome AIDS. Not everyone who has HIV has AIDS, but everyone who has AIDS has HIV.

Illness Behavior occurs when a decision is made by the client to determine whether to seek medical care and what type of care to seek. The decision is usually based on the type and severity of symptoms experienced.

Indicators are measures that reflect the condition of a system.

Infectious Diseases are diseases that can be passed from one person to another by various means such as sputum, blood, body secretions, airborne mucous particles etc. Examples of infectious diseases include pneumonia, hepatitis, HIV, and tuberculosis.

Informed Consent is designed to protect people and institutions from any harm, experimentation, or exploitation. It is the voluntary agreement to participate in a study by individuals or agencies after they have received a complete explanation of the purpose, procedures and risks and gains involved, and have understood the explanation.

Internet is a global network of computers. Originally designed by the United States Department of Defense (DOD) to permit information sharing among institutions working on DOD projects, the Internet is now available to anyone with a computer.

Internet Service Provider is an organization or company that provides access to the public Internet.

Key Informants are information-rich providers and users of health care services who are recognized as having experience or expertise with a specific issue, and can provide valuable information and insights into the needs of a community or a specific group within the community.

Key Stakeholders are those individuals responsible for the development and administration of mental health services provided to children, adults, and families within agencies providing services to specified regions and populations

Leading Health Indicators are ten attributes, such as tobacco use, or physical activity, that reflect the nation's health and wellness concerns.

They are used in *Healthy People 2010* to predict future trends in health and wellness status and behaviors. They were selected by a work group formed by the agencies of the U.S. Department of Health and Human Services. In health assessment, Leading Health Indicators provide baseline data on health behaviors.

Low Birth Weight (LBW) refers to a newborn that weighs less than 2500 grams at birth, which is approximately five and one-half pounds.

Mental Disorders are difficult to define succinctly. A disorder is comprised of a myriad of complex signs and symptoms that are interpreted based upon varied levels of abstraction and influencing concepts. Clinical definitions represent disorders as clinically significant behavioral or psychological syndromes or patterns. Health is altered in changes that occur to mood, behavior, and thoughts either singularly or in various combinations. The disorder may be perceived by the affected individual and associated with distress, disability, suffering, death, pain, or losses of freedom. Conversely, the individual may not have full awareness, understanding, or insight into the presenting health problem. A disorder can occur in males or females of any age, race, or ethnic group. Family histories, genetics, biological, environmental, social, or behavioral factors that occur independently or in combination have been attributed to the development of mental disorders.

Mental Health is defined by each individual according to actual or perceived satisfaction with his or her level of psychological functioning, or according to prevailing or influencing sociocutural standards.

Mental Health Services include interventions for prevention, diagnosis, and treatment. In general, services are geared toward supporting and improving an individual's coping with those issues that threaten maintenance of mental health or improve physical, emotional, and social functioning when mental illness is present.

Mental Illness is a general term often used as a collective reference to any diagnosable mental disorder.

Multisystem Disease Process is a myriad of diseases in which more than one organ or body system is affected. This is due to the interrelationships of the malfunctioning organ with other organs involved in the diagnosis of one disease.

Node is a part of a URL. At the highest level (the left side of the URL), these parts of a URL are separated by periods (dot com, for example) and identify a particular computer on the Internet. At lower levels, the nodes are separated by slashes (/), and identify a directory or directory structure on a disk drive on a computer.

Normative Needs are the benchmarks described by *Healthy People 2010*. They are recognized standards for health outcomes for population groups in the aggregate.

Objectives are developed from the general goal, and support the general goal. They are more specifically worded goals that can be measured over a specified period of time to evaluate the progress of the plan. *Healthy People 2010's* 467 objectives are all designed to support its 28 goals.

Outcomes are often distinguished from outputs (i.e., units of service, conformance to specifications, satisfaction, and timeliness).

"Immediate" outcomes refer to cognitive and affective change. "Intermediate" outcomes refer to behavioral change. "Long-term" outcomes refer to improved life chances or improved "quality of life."

Parity is a term pertaining to equity within health care insurance. Benefits as well as limitations of health care insurance coverage under medical, surgical, mental illness, and mental health services would be unbiased. The presence of full parity coverage would prevent discrimination based upon a diagnosis of a mental disorder or upon an individual seeking mental health services.

Preconceptual Planning is a process of actively planning for the conception, pregnancy, and birth, incorporating the three components of health promotion, risk assessment, and proper treatment (WAPC, 2000).

Prenatal refers to the period of time from conception to labor.

Preterm birth is one occurring before 37th weeks of gestation. Full term is 40 weeks' gestation.

Primary health care is the point of health care service where consumers first enter the health care system. For child-bearing women, this might be the obstetrician/gynecologist; for a young child, primary health care would first begin at the pediatrician, or pediatric nurse practitioner.

QSR NVivo is a software program that analyzes qualitative data.

Quality of Life is a generic term that has been used in developing some community-based indicators reports. Unlike two other organizing principles—*Healthy People* and the concept of sustainability—broad

agreement on its meaning has not yet been achieved.

Request for Proposal (RFP) is a request for proposals that may be issued by a community coalition as part of an action plan.

Resilience is a personal trait or characteristic that contributes to an individual's ability to develop coping resources, adapt, and become competent in managing the stressors of life (U.S. Department of Health and Human Services, 1999).

Scientific Method is a systematic step-by-step process of conducting research.

Search Engine is a program used to locate data on the Internet. Examples are AltaVista, Googol, HotBot, and Yahoo!

Secondary Health Care is treatment of a disease process in the acute phase. This might include something as simple as taking prescribed medications to halt temporarily or eliminate the progression of a disease process.

Self-Extracting Archive is a compressed file that has been modified so that it can be executed like a program. Executing or running the file results in the uncompressed file being extracted from the archive file.

Serious Mental Illness (SMI) is a chronic mental illness usually found in persons age 18 and older. However, many mental illnesses have their onset in childhood or adolescence and some are identified retrospectively in early adult years. Nevertheless, the individual is severely affected throughout life and experiences serious limitations and challenges the ability to function in life and society.

Service Learning refers to "a method of teaching through which students apply newly acquired academic skills and knowledge to address real-life needs in their own communities" (Payne, 2000, pp. 3–4).

Social Support is the feeling of being cared for by others.

Spina Bifida is a congenital defect at the lower end of the spinal column that may result in varying degrees of physical impairment, including paralysis below the waist with loss of bowel and bladder control.

Spreadsheet is a file containing data that can be viewed and analyzed in a program such as Microsoft Excel. A spreadsheet organizes data into columns and rows with a row representing one case and a column representing one datum per case. Each cell in a spreadsheet can contain data, a label, or a formula.

Sponsor is a term that refers to an individual, organization, or coalition that issues an invitation to a meeting for the purpose of developing a community-based indicators report and intervention initiative. Sponsors often provide the resources that sustain an indicators initiative through its formative steps.

SPSS (Statistical Package for the Social Sciences) is a software program that analyzes quantitative data.

Steering Committee refers to the team that selects the principle(s) that will guide the development of an indicators initiative, develops a selection criteria, and chooses the indicators with respect to which data will be gathered.

Strong Democracy is a term coined by Benjamin Barber. It refers to "politics in the participatory mode, where conflict is resolved in the absence of an independent ground through a participatory process of

ongoing, proximate self-legislation, and the creation of a political community capable of transforming dependent, private individuals into free citizens, and partial and private interests into public goods" (1984, p. 132).

Structured Query Language (SQL) is the language of modern databases. It is used to request data meeting your requirements from the database.

Survey is a means by which researchers gather sample data from a generalizable population.

Sustainability refers to "an evolving process that improves the economy, the environment, and society for the benefit of current and future generations" (President's Council on Sustainable Development, 1996). Sustainability has been used as a guiding principle in the development of community-based indicators.

Sustainable Development refers to a program that can be used to "change the process of economic development so that it can ensure a basic quality of life for all people while protecting ecosystems and community systems that make life possible and worthwhile" (International Council for Local Economic Initiatives, 1996).

Table is the basic storage method of a database. As displayed, it resembles a spreadsheet. It differs from a spreadsheet in that a cell can only contain data or the results of a formula that is applied to every cell in a column. A similar structure on a web page can actually hold anything that can be placed on a web page. In this case it is a convenient structure for organizing data for presentation rather than a method for storing large amounts of data.

Target population is a group within a community, or a group within several communities that share a given concern or attribute. For instance, all pregnant women, regardless of ethnic origin or community location, share the need to access adequate prenatal care in the first trimester of pregnancy.

Tertiary Health Care addresses events taken to limit the course of a disease process. An example might be a client undergoing coronary artery bypass graft surgery due to blockage of the coronary arteries.

Uniform Resource Locator (URL), also commonly referred to as a web address, is a string of characers that uniquely identifies a file on the Internet.

Very Low Birth Weight (VLBW) refers to infants who weigh less than 1500 grams at birth (slightly more than 3 pounds).

Web Page is a file that contains Hypertext Markup Language (HTML) and may also contain references to other files that will be displayed at a computer in a web browser program such as Internet Explorer or Netscape Navigator.

Web Site is a collection of web pages connected with each other by HTML references.

Wellness refers to quality of life, a general satisfaction in all of the areas of an individual's life, including aesthetic, cultural, educational. economic, emotional, environmental, mental, physical, relational, and spiritual.

WIC (Women, Infants and Children) is a federally funded, state-administered food assistance program offering nutrition assistance to pregnant and breastfeeding women, infants, and children up to age 5.

World Wide Web is an information retrieval system using Hypertext to present information from the Internet. Until the introducton of the web in 1991, internet access was strictly character-based and command driven.